Drainage and Sanitation

Rolf Payne

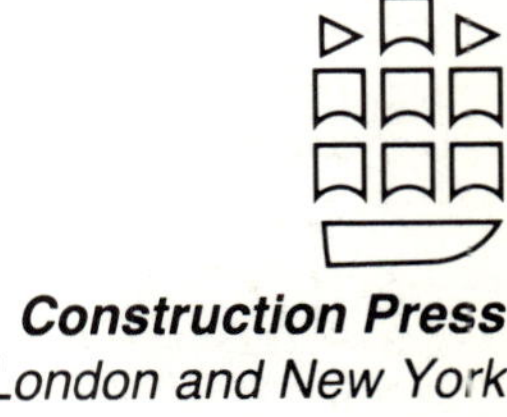

Construction Press
London and New York

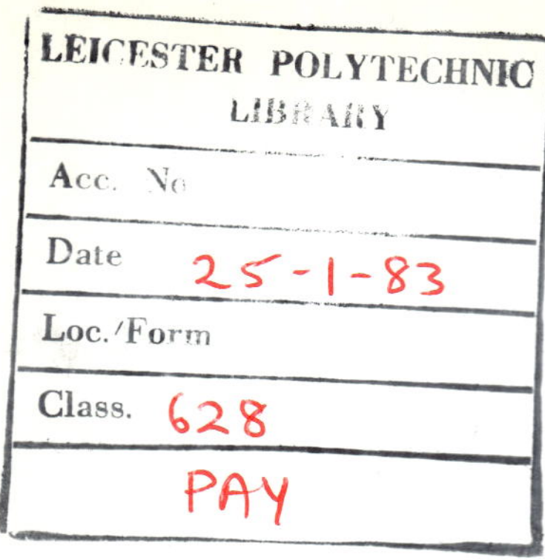

General Editor: Colin Bassett, BSc, FCIOB, FFB

Construction Press
Longman House
Burnt Mill, Harlow, Essex, UK

A division of Longman Group Limited, London

Published in the United States of America
by Longman Inc., New York

First published 1982

British Library Cataloguing in Publication Data

Payne, Rolf
Drainage and sanitation
1. Sanitary engineering
I. Title
628 TD145

ISBN 0-582-41241-2

Library of Congress Cataloging in Publication Data

Payne, Rolf, 1928–
Drainage and sanitation.

Includes index.
1. Drainage, House. 2. Sanitary engineering.
I. Title
TH6571.P393 696'.13 82-1455
ISBN 0-582-41241-2 AACR2

Printed in Great Britain at The Pitman Press, Bath

Contents

Acknowledgements

We are grateful to the following for permission to reproduce copyright material: Fig. 2.1, Marley Extrusions Ltd., photographers Geo P. King Ltd.; Fig. 2.2, Associated Metal Works Glasgow Ltd; Fig. 2.3 (redrawn from material provided) and 2.5, Armitage Shanks Ltd; Fig. 2.4, the Regional Architect, Oxford Regional Health Authority; Fig. 2.8, C. E. Wardell & Hesp; Fig. 4.5, British Industrial Plastics Limited, photographers Turners Photography Ltd; Fig. 4.8, Chris Haigh Photographics; Fig. 5.8, David Whiting Photography; Fig. 4.11, 9.1, 11.3, 11.8, Crown copyright, reproduced by permission of the Controller of Her Majesty's Stationery Office; Figs. 7.12 and 8.8, Harley Extrusions Ltd; Table 8.3, Athlone (contracting) Ltd; Figs. 8.5 and 8.6, Sigmund Pulsometer Pumps Ltd; Fig. 8.11, A. F. Trenchers Ltd; Fig. 8.14, Althon (contracting) Ltd; Fig. 11.8, Wards Flexible Rod Co. Ltd.

Information provided in the Agrément certificate is reproduced by permission of Verkstads AB Durgo, Solna, Sweden.

Chapter 1

Introduction

The objective of this publication is to provide those people interested in the design, installation and management of drainage systems some guidance information based upon the author's own experiences in research, design practice and maintenance; it is intended to be a guide to good practice.

In the text I refer to 'drainage'. The word is meant to be all-embracing and covers all sanitary pipework systems from the point of discharge from an appliance to the outfall or treatment plant.

In our sophisticated twentieth century Western society we tend to take for granted many aspects of our standard of living such as motorways, aeroplanes, medical care, pure water and flush sanitation that inhabitants of other countries and indeed our grandparents would know little about.

If we look back less than two generations it was unusual to find internal sanitation in our buildings, but about 1830 sewers were beginning to be constructed and public health was considered an advanced science by community-minded officials.

Acceleration in the installation of sanitary systems occurred between 1830 and 1866, and was mainly due to the increase in cholera within our city complexes and the linking of the disease to unsanitary conditions. In London it was recommended that Parliament should be moved away from the River Thames because of the appalling smell from this open sewer.

During 1849, over 14 000 people died from cholera in London alone and again in 1858 10 000 were laid low from this killer disease. It must also be remembered that the population of our capital city in this period of our history was only a few millions.

In 1936 the government brought together various regulations and local codes of practice, etc., into one comprehensive Public Health Act of Parliament which deals with the whole question of 'Sanitation in Buildings' (Part II).

When complemented by the Building Regulations (often revised) and various British Standards and BS Codes of Practice (always out of date) these documents form the basis of our present-day high standard of sanitary engineering.

In the United Kingdom the fundamental design concept of our drainage systems relies upon the force of gravity to remove the waste solids discharged with water through sanitary appliances from the point of discharge to the place of treatment. This system requires therefore a gradient for near horizontal pipework systems whether they are below ground or slung in service voids within a building. It is therefore vitally important that nothing impedes the free flow of the effluent, causing stoppages to occur.

The pumping of effluent and surface water can and is undertaken when necessary, but it is expensive in both equipment and maintenance costs and should be avoided if at all possible.

The drainage of the sanitary appliances in vertical buildings such as high-rise blocks of flats is by the use of vertical stacks (pipes) throughout the height of the building, and therefore the grouping of the appliances around the stacks is of considerable importance if we do not wish to complicate the systems. It is particularly important that each individual dwelling has a self-contained system within the dwelling, only joining into a common vertical stack before discharging into a communal underground system.

A well-designed and correctly installed sanitary system that is not outrageously misused should and will function for many years without attention; indeed, 'out of sight, out of mind' is a typical attitude to this important service, well founded upon user experience.

Systems will, however, deteriorate with age and will fail if misused – by which is meant they will become blocked and cease to function as the user required and the designer intended. It is therefore important that from time to time the complete systems are checked and maintenance undertaken before failure occurs.

The traditional approach to design techniques applied to drainage systems has grown and developed over the years with little regard to science or research. Only in the past twenty-five years has research been carried out by various organizations, and in particular the Building Research Establishment, Watford, to provide design and installation information based on hydraulic considerations. Much of this information is published in Digests and Current Papers which have been freely used in this publication.

Obviously conflict arises between traditionalists and those attempting to apply design advice based upon research.

The approach used in this publication is based upon research, coupled with a large dose of practical design, installation and estate management experience. But at no time does it blindly follow the 'rule of thumb', which so often cannot be adapted successfully to systems required for more complex developments than housing, such as hospitals and industrial estates.

In our cost-conscious society we have to draw a fine line between good design and the cost of the job. This has also been taken into account, but at no time will the cost influence the design to a degree when the system will become unsafe.

It must always be at the back of the mind of the designer that if failure of a drainage system occurs there is a risk to health due to the possible release of pathogenic, corrosive or even radio-active effluent into the environment.

Chapter 2

Appliances

Introduction

We are all familiar with domestic sanitary appliances – sinks, basins, baths and WCs – and this chapter is not intended to be a catalogue of items, but to bring to the attention of specifiers, designers and maintenance managers the part appliances play in the operation of sanitary pipework systems.

As well as the well-known appliances I have included traps, gullies and wastes, and also those special pieces of equipment that can affect the performance of the drainage system.

All effluents start their journey through the drainage system from sanitary appliances or special equipment connected to the pipework system.

There are two broad types of appliances, those that are used for the disposal of waste products where cold water is used as the conveying medium, and those appliances which are used for washing or cleaning purposes where water at various temperatures is used combined with cleaning agents such as soap or detergents when, therefore, the amount of conveyed solids is small.

The function of the appliance dictates the solid-to-liquid relationship and quantity of the effluent discharged, all of which is of considerable importance if we are to design pipework systems that will not fail, or create a nuisance by being noisy, or allow smells to penetrate our buildings.

The objective of all appliances is therefore to provide the user – or abuser – with convenient disposal points for either unwanted waste products, or for waste cleaning liquids.

Variability of use

Each and every appliance will be used at a different time of the day or night, for a varying number and length of time, and will discharge effluents of varying quality, quantity and consistency.

In effect the times and amounts are the controlling factors which dictate the size and gradient of the drainage system; we tend to disregard the solid content. We are therefore interested in the quantity, frequency of use and length of time sanitary appliances discharge so that we can design successfully. The overlap of the discharges from different appliances builds up the flow in the pipework system until we obtain continuous flow in our sewers.

Numerous tests and measurements from a variety of domestic appliances have been made and recorded; these also include public buildings and offices, but not hospitals. Table 2.1 gives the relationships for some standard sanitary appliances.

Table 2.1 Quantities and flows from appliances (data from BS 5572 and BRE technical literature)

Appliance	*Quantity in litres*	*Max. flow in l/sec.*	*Duration of flow in sec.*	*Frequency between uses in seconds*
Washdown WC	9	2.3	5	1200 600 300
Urinal (single units)	4.5	0.15	30	1200 900
Basin	6	0.6	10	1200 600 300
Sink	23	0.9	25	1200 600 300
Bath	80	1.1	75	4500 1800
Automatic washing machine	180	0.7	300	1500
Shower	—	0.1	—	—
Spray tap	—	0.06	—	—

Water closet cisterns usually discharge 9 litres in about 5 seconds, but dual flush cisterns are now being increasingly specified as standard. These cisterns can be made to discharge either 9 litres or 4.5 litres, depending upon the requirement of the user.

The objective of providing dual flush cisterns is solely to save water. It has been found by experience that because of the inadequate self-cleansing flush provided by 4.5 litres an increasing number of blockages are occurring within our drainage systems, particularly those that are installed in rough bore materials such as cast iron.

Only where the WC user is educated to accept and understand the function of the two types of discharge should they be specified.

It must be noted that certain capacities (litres) given in the table will vary dependent upon certain physical aspects of the appliance, i.e. a small basin often fitted in a WC compartment will hold less than a large basin in a wash room. The rate of discharge will also, in *l*/sec., vary between basis of the same capacity depending upon the funnel shape from the rim down to the waste outlet; the velocity of the discharge will increase or decrease depending upon this shape.

Appliances such as baths and sinks with flat bottoms have a slow end discharge that will fill the trap.

Traps and wastes

Coupled with all appliances, sometimes as an integral part of the appliance (such as a WC) or as close to the equipment as is possible, is a water-filled sealed trap. The only purpose of an appliance trap is to prevent foul air within the sewers and drains from entering our buildings. It is not – as some would have us think – to prevent rats from entering our buildings, as tests and observations have shown that rats can easily swim through a water-sealed trap of adequate size.

A trap in itself can be a discharge point into the drainage system; a typical example being a kitchen floor gully used as a disposal point for floor washings.

The type and shape of the waste outlet does not unduly affect the rate of discharge from an appliance, but the type and shape of the trap will do so. There are effective differences between the rate of flow from a 'P', 'S' or bottle type trap.

Minimum sizes of tubular traps are given in BS 5572 table 4, and it is usual to specify bottle traps of the same diameter waste and outlet.

There is a general move by designers away from the traditional metal 'P' or 'S' type trap to the plastic bottle trap. This is usually because of the relative ease of maintenance of a bottle trap by removing the trap bowl and emptying the contents; it is also easier to hide a bottle trap behind the pedestal of a basin.

The decision to use bottle traps throughout a building for all appliances

Table 2.2 Minimum size of traps (data from BS 5572 and BRE technical literature)

Appliance	*Trap size*
Wash Basins Bidet Drinking fountain	32 mm
Sink Bath Shower tray Sink with disposal unit Urinal	40 mm
Industrial waste disposal unit Bedpan macerator Sanitary towel macerator	50 mm
WC Slophoppers Sluices	100 mm

Note: Some WCs can discharge into a 75 mm stack or branch depending upon the internal bore of the trap.

should not be lightly taken as certain discharges from appliances such as macerators and sinks may quickly block this type of trap. They should never be used for bedpan disposal units.

Materials

Traditionally sanitary appliances such as WCs and basins are manufactured in vitreous china, although plastics, fireclay and stainless steel are also used.

When choosing the appliance the material of manufacture should be considered. It is important that the appliance is both hydraulically and physically suitable for the function intended and that it will not deteriorate or become easily damaged.

Vitreous china

This is a white clay body which is vitrified in a continuous kiln and permanently fused with a vitreous glazed surface which may be white or coloured. It is proof against rot, stains and burning, is rustless, non-fading and resistant to acids and alkalis. It has a 99.5 per cent vitreosity which ensures that even unglazed it cannot be contaminated by bacteria. It is also very hard wearing and does not craze.

Fireclay

Usually used for the manufacture of large items such as shower trays, stall urinals, washing troughs, etc. The fireclay is covered with a white or coloured vitreous ceramic glaze and may be proof against crazing.

Such items are heavy and are now manufactured in other materials such as plastics or stainless steel.

Plastics

A variety of plastics are used for the manufacture of sanitary appliances and it is important that before selecting the appliance on shape and colour the material should be investigated, and also the support system, as plastics are usually not structurally strong.

They are used in the manufacture of baths, basins and shower trays.

'Plastic' is a relatively soft material and can be easily burnt or scratched. It also has greater thermal movement than traditional materials and therefore the sealing of the joint between fixed surfaces such as partitions and the appliance is important to prevent the ingress of water and the growth of bacteria.

Appliances made in plastic are lighter in weight and usually cost less than their more traditional counterpart.

Most manufacturers' literature states that you should not use abrasive powder

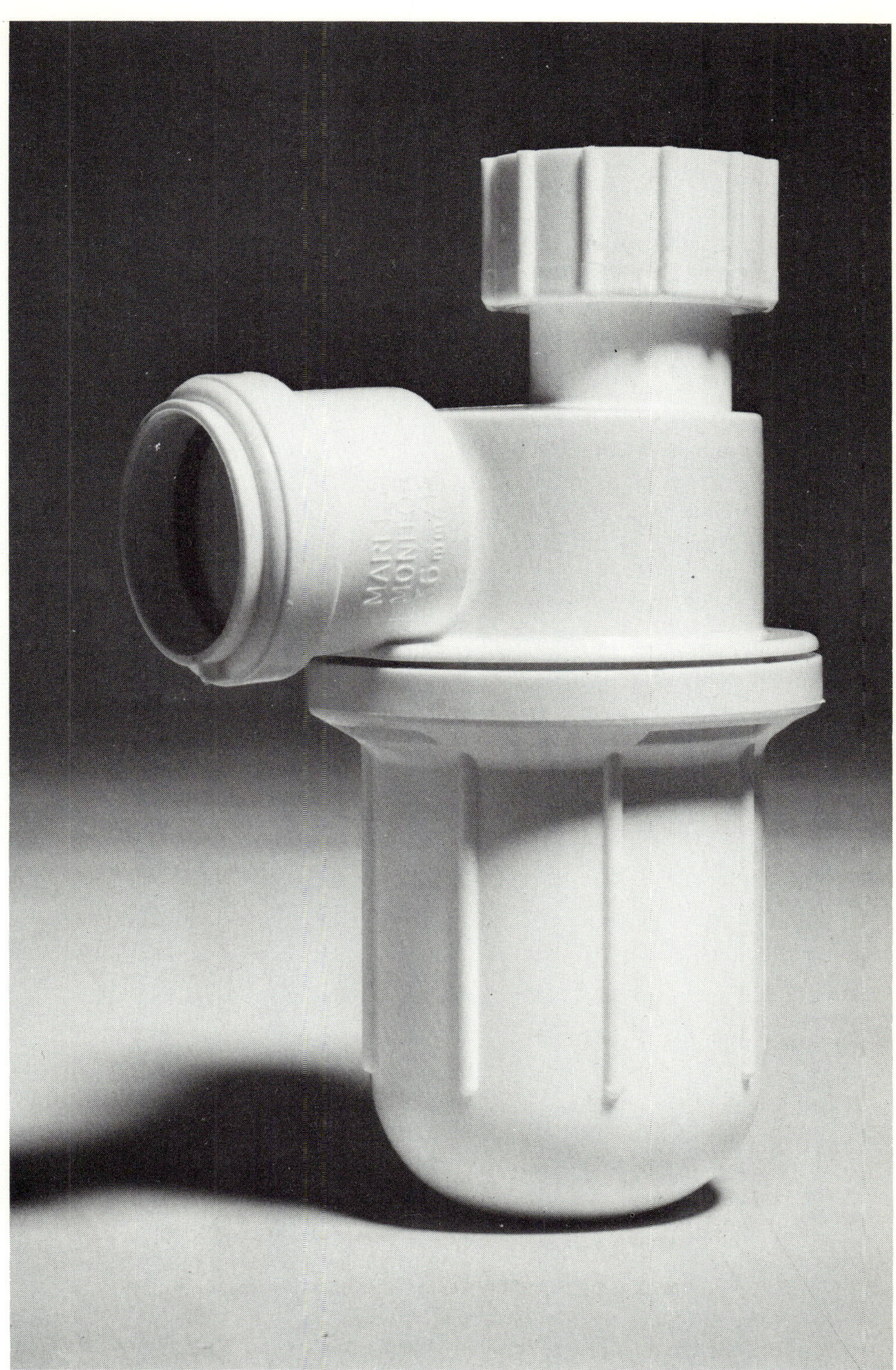

Fig. 2.1 Bottle resealing trap

cleaners and that slight scratches can be polished out – giving an indication of the life expectancy in terms of appearance, and possible maintenance requirements.

Steel

Only baths, shower trays and vanity basins are now manufactured in pressed steel coated with a vitreous enamel finish which may be easily chipped if an object is dropped on to the surface. Once the integratory of the surface is broken rusting will quickly start if immediate maintenance is not undertaken. It has been noted that crazing sometimes occurs around the waste outlet.

Cast iron

This is traditionally used for the manufacture of baths, which are then stove enamelled which provides a high-gloss, impervious finish resistant to acids and alkalis and capable of giving years of service.

Obviously very heavy and difficult to manoeuvre upstairs.

Stainless steel

Used for the manufacture of many types of sanitary appliances, particularly for

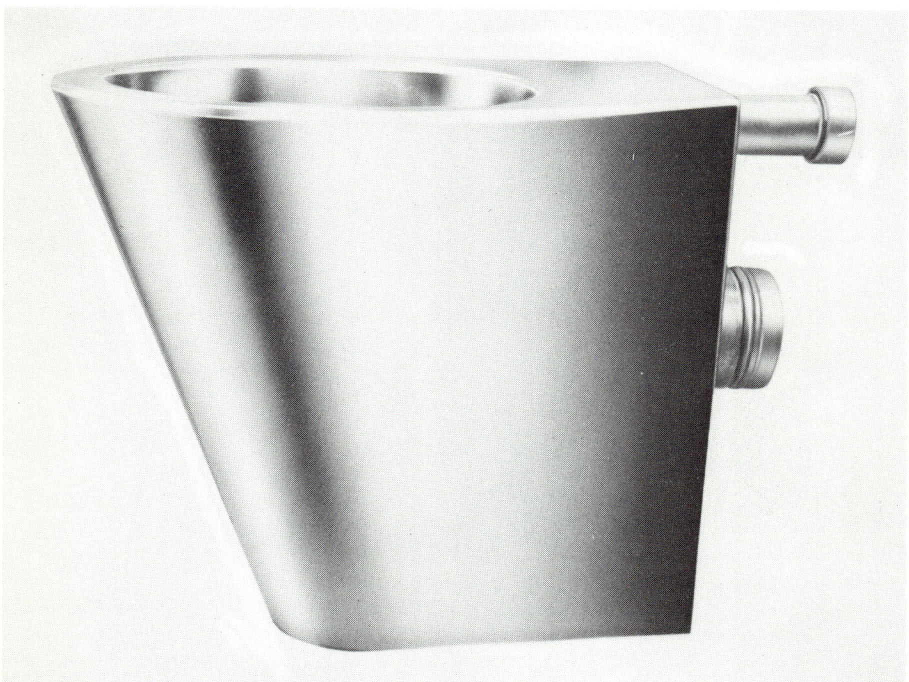

Fig. 2.2 Stainless steel WC

the catering industry, laboratories and hospitals; also where vandalism is likely as it does not shatter as will vitreous china.

Sink tops are manufactured in stainless steel, but basins and WCs are also available.

Stainless steel can be made to a number of formulations, but is usually of low carbon 18 per cent chromium, 10 per cent nickel, or when an increased resistance to hot strong acetic acids are required 3 per cent molybdenum is added.

Preplumbed units

Where repetitive sanitary appliances and accommodation is to be used throughout a large building or number of similar buildings such as hospitals or hotels, consideration should be given to the use of some type of standard preplumbed unit.

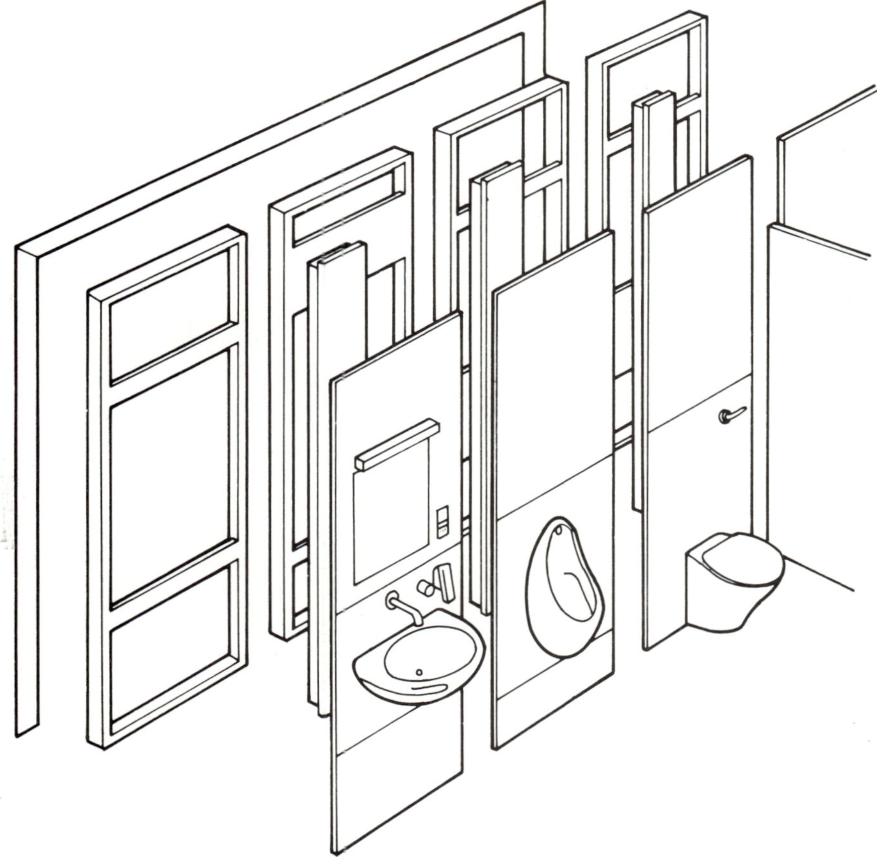

Fig. 2.3 Typical preplumbed unit (permission Armitage)

Most sanitary ware manufacturers provide such units modulely co-ordinated and capable of being assembled in various configurations. This method of erection and installation forestalls any damage during the general construction on site. Because they are factory manufactured the standard of finish and construction can usually be improved and the installation left until the wet trades have finished.

Health care appliances

Regional Health Authorities often use standard products and assemblies to

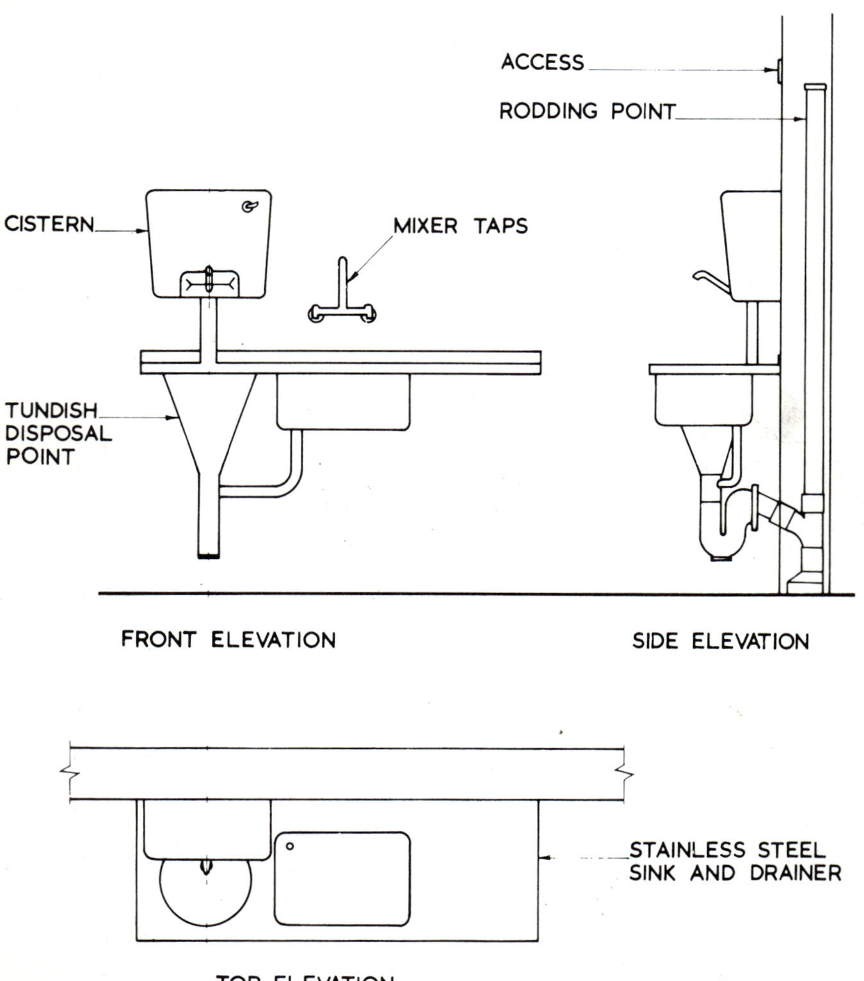

Fig. 2.4 Oxford Regional Health Authority standard sanitary assembly

reduce the time required to select these items for each project. This releases architects and designers to concentrate on the building rather than small items of equipment.

The Department of Health and Social Security in collaboration with manufacturers and the Regional Health Authorities have issued guidance and information on clinically acceptable standard items of sanitary ware, suitable for use in health care buildings. In general there is a performance standard laid down and this covers appliances to British Standards; only white is specified, with a diffused brightness factor of not less than 85 per cent. It states that the finish and shape of all sanitary ware should be streamlined for ease of cleaning, with junctions and ledges eliminated as far as possible.

The hospital WC (often now used in hotels) is of the rimless type, fixed to the floor and back to the wall, and the seat is designed for easy removal for cleaning purposes. Various tests are specified and detailed information is given by the manufacturers' Product Specification and by the DHSS in their Manufacturer's Data Bank (MDB) publications.

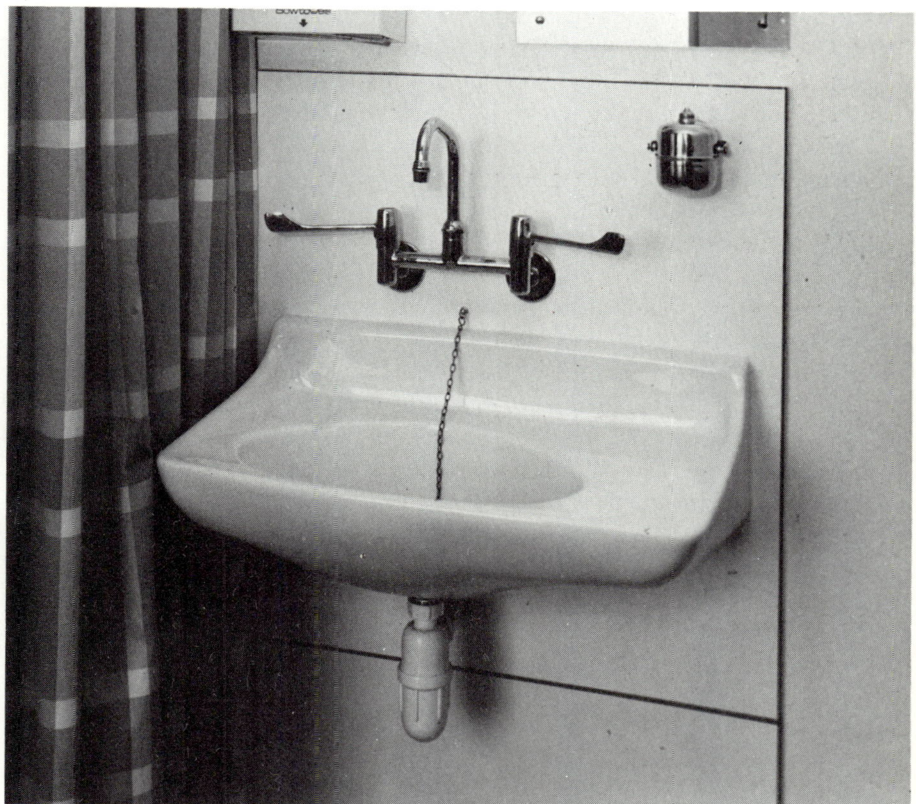

Fig. 2.5 Hospital basin

It will be noted that chain stay holes and overflows are omitted from the specification for the standard range of basins, and that in a number of cases taps have also been removed from the appliance and wall mounted. The object is to remove dirt catchment points and orifices where bacteria can breed.

It is also advised that baths used for clinical purposes should not be supplied with overflows as bathing often forms part of the medical treatment of the patient.

Special equipment

Some items of equipment are specifically discussed as they have special effects on the drainage system, usually requiring changes in design or materials.

Many of the items are specific to hospitals, laboratories or kitchens.

Macerators

Free standing or sink-fitted macerators are used for the convenient disposal, via the drainage system, of biodegradable solids. It is a quick, hygienic method of disposal if properly used, but before specifying such units it must be ascertained that the pipework and sewer system is capable of taking the load.

The units may be a small domestic model or large industrial units used in commercial kitchens or laboratories.

The waste effluent may be pathogenic.

Solids are fed into the machines with running cold water, and because it is a convenient dustbin the effluent can cause serious blockages within the pipework system. Dry bread, cellulose and starch products may cause blockages if macerated in bulk, as they swell when wet.

It is very important that the pipework associated with all types of macerator or waste disposal unit is of smooth bore, the joints of which are flush and the fittings well radiused.

Plastic is an ideal material for this system.

The waste pipes should be short, not exceeding 3 m, and installed at a gradient of not less than 1 in 50.

There must be an access point near to the unit at the head of the system and if possible the effluent should discharge into a stack or drain carrying a good flow from other appliances.

Under no circumstances should any macerator discharge into a gully or interceptor.

Bedpan disposal units

These units are specifically designed macerators for the disposal of papier-mache bedpans and urinal bottles. The items are placed in the units prior to maceration, which takes place to a timed cycle with cold water. The effluent is then flushed out of the unit as a pulverized pulp waste into the drainage system. The papier-mache consistency is regulated by the automatic water supply and the number of items placed in the unit – the maximum acceptable being stated by the unit manufacturers. If this number is exceeded the effluent consistency will form a thick porridge which may block the waste pipe from the machine and/or the drainage pipework, particularly if the system is in cast iron.

It is important that the designer or specifier should ensure that the drainage system of any building is capable of taking this type of effluent.

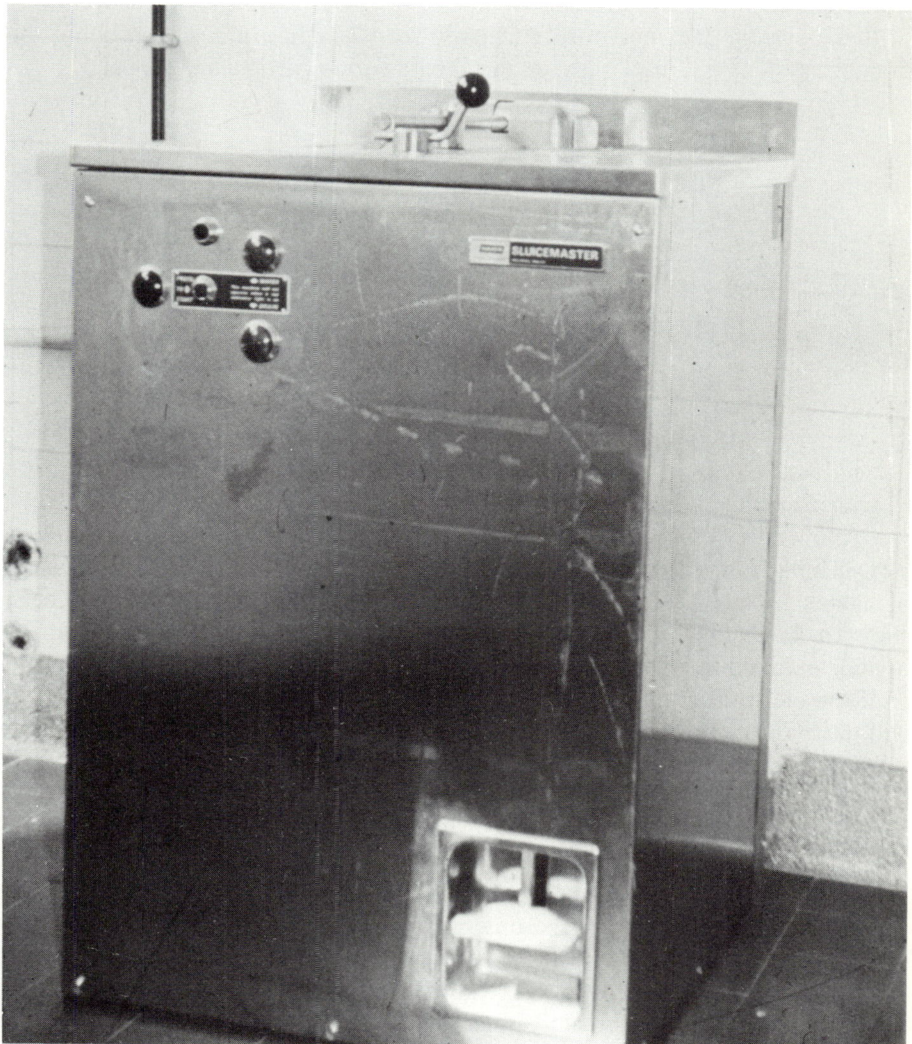

Fig. 2.6 Bedpan disposal unit

Silver recovery unit

These units are used in photographic and X-ray processing to recover the silver washed out in the developing processes.

Two basic types of equipment are used:

(a) Metal exchange.
(b) Electrolitic.

The metal exchange system relies upon the silver being deposited on to steel wool pads by the reaction of the noble metal (silver) on the base metal (steel) in which the silver replaces the steel wool.

If the system does not work efficiently the waste liquid discharged into the drainage system will react with the metal pipework – particularly copper.

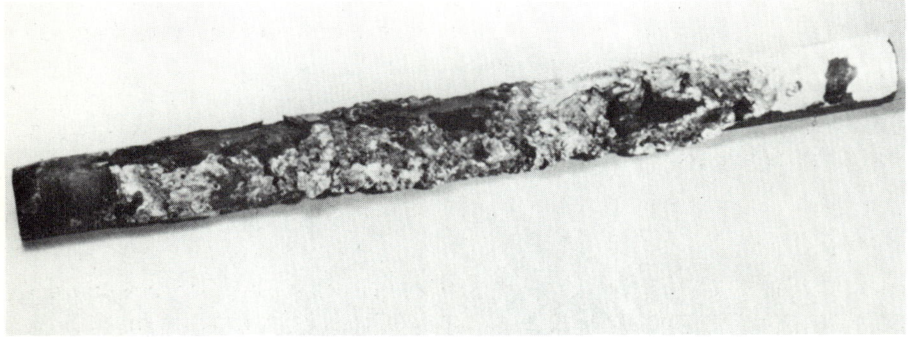

Fig. 2.7 Section of copper waste from Silver Recovery Unit

Deposits from the process may be carried through into the drains, causing blockages by a brown glutinous plastic material which, on analysis, has been shown to be 25 to 30 per cent organic matter (ferruginous bacteria), the main inorganic matter being gesthite (oxide of iron).

If the electrolitic processing equipment fails the photographic fixing solution will enter the drainage system and may cause damage to the sewage treatment work; it may also contravene the Public Health Act 1936, Section 27.

Equipment using chemicals

Various chemicals are used in industrial and hospital analytical equipment and the designer must investigate those items where he is unsure of the composition or reaction of the effluents upon the pipework, maintenance operators and treatment works. Expert advice may be required.

One commonly used chemical is sodium azide which is a cheap, soluble and effective preservative, and provided it does not come into contact with heavy metals such as copper, lead, brass and zinc – all used in drainage systems – it can be used with safety. If it does contact these metals metallic azide crystals are formed which are powerful explosives, sensitive to shock, friction or heat. Copper azide in particular is very unstable and will detonate with the slightest mechanical shock.

Certain chemicals, although innocuous in themselves, become dangerous when mixed in the drainage system with other chemicals. It is advisable therefore when working on the design of laboratory drainage systems to check carefully all equipment and processes being specified, as separate networks may be necessary.

Many chemicals in relatively small quantities may be disposed of via the drainage system, including dilute radioactive liquids. As chemicals and laboratory techniques are changing constantly we do not know what is likely to enter the system in time to come, consequently we must design particularly to chemical drainage standards, because however careful the user may be it is always likely that a spillage may occur of a quantity of a chemical which would require quickly washing down the nearest drain.

A douche shower should be installed in all laboratories.

Drainage systems for laboratories must be in chemically inert materials, the best of which is glass.

Dishwashers and washing machines

Domestic dishwashers and washing machines will in no way affect a good drainage system, and may in fact help in keeping it clean and in good condition.

One effect that may cause trouble is the excess foaming of detergents which may block a stack or drain, thereby preventing the free movement of air throughout the system.

Industrial machines should not discharge into plastic drainage systems because the continuous flow of very hot water can cause softening and collapse of the material. Copper, clay ware or spun iron should be used.

Siphonic WCs

This type of WC is clinically more acceptable than the wash down type as the flushing action does not create such an aerosol with consequently, a lower risk of bacterial contamination of body organs.

They are, however, more liable to blockages within the syphon, and should not therefore be specified for situations where they are liable to become receptacles for paper towels or other 'disposable' products. They are particularly not suitable for maternity or psychiatric units.

Shower trays and foot baths

These items of equipment usually sit on the floor surface and the trap is either in, or directly under, the floor. Consequently if the trap becomes blocked it is a difficult operation to clear it.

The choice of waste outlet is important and they are now available with removable grilles to enable easy access through the clear bore waste into the trap. Only 'P' or 'S' type traps should be used.

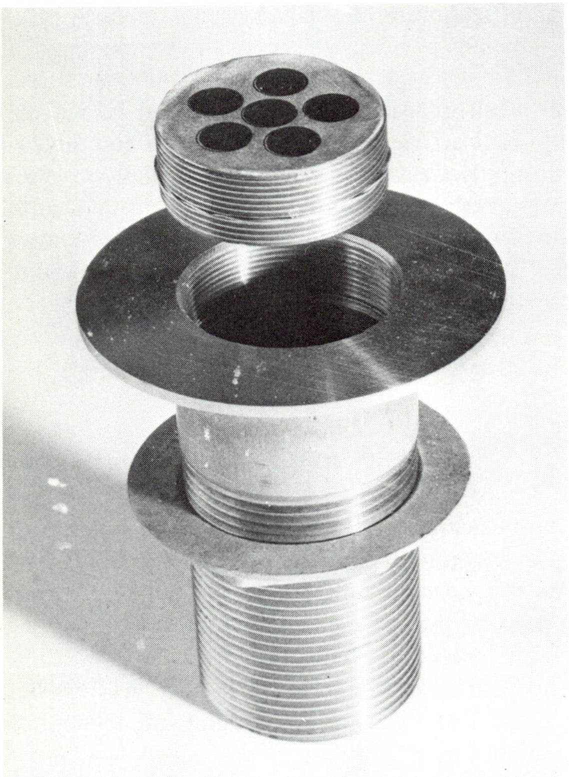

Fig. 2.8 Clear bore waste outlet

The particular model illustrated in Fig. 2.8 has the facility that the removed grille can be reversed to take a standing waste which turns a shower tray into a foot bath.

Spray taps and showers

These are used under very different circumstances, but their effect on the drainage system is similar. They both provide a small quantity of water for washing purposes, and because of the low flow the water, when combined with soap, dirt and body particles such as dead skin and hair, can allow sedimentation to occur within the pipework and a slow blockage will develop. It is therefore advisable to restrict the length of waste to under 4 m and provide a gradient of not less than 1 in 50. Access is provided if the clear bore waste is used, but a cleansing flush into the drain from another appliance such as a bath or WC is recommended.

Planned maintenance may be necessary.

Bidets

These are often referred to as sit-on wash basins; they are also sometimes used as foot baths.

It is important to ensure that the water supply conforms with the requirements of the Water Authority and there is no risk of back siphonage occurring.

In certain circumstances bidets and showers may become soil appliances when used by incontinent persons who may accidentally evacuate themselves when using the equipment. This may happen in geriatric accommodation and it is important that the trap, and pipework, should be capable of taking the effluent without blocking. Only 'P' or 'S' type traps should be used.

Plaster sinks and slophoppers

Both these items of equipment may, if not correctly used, allow the ingress into the system of objects likely to cause blockages.

It is important that plaster sink sediment receivers or lift-out wire screens do not allow plaster to enter the system; likewise the cleaning staff must not discharge through slophoppers mop heads, cleaning cloths or other items that will cause blockages.

This is a management function requiring the education of the users who must be made aware of the problems they can cause by the misuse or poor maintenance of equipment.

Post mortem and dissecting tables

During the use and subsequent cleaning of this equipment small parts of body tissue and body fluids are likely to enter the drainage system.

Formalin or other chemicals may also be discharged.

There are two consequences from these actions:

(a) that fat particles may block the trap and pipework system; they may be pathogenic;

(b) the formalin or other chemical vapour may collect under the manhole or access covers and become released during maintenance operations.

It is important that all the pipework connected to this type of equipment is of smooth bore and installed to a very high standard.

Double trapping should not be used and it is preferable that the equipment trap is sited next to the tables and maintained by the laboratory staff.

The general drain maintenance staff must be informed of those drains likely to contain pathogenic or chemical waste and instructed in the correct procedures to operate when working on the system.

Where there is a likelihood of dangerous vapours collecting additional ventilation pipework should be provided.

Chapter 3

Types of drainage

Introduction

A debate that often occupies the time of people interested in drainage is the difference between 'sewerage', 'drainage', 'foul', 'soil' and 'waste' systems, trade effluent, rainwater, surface and storm water.

The various Codes and Regulations give Definitions or Interpretations of these terms, but as far as the designer is concerned they all mean about the same and can be simplified to three basic systems; the names are irrelevant except as a means of communication.

Foul sewerage or soil drainage systems

These convey any waste contaminated by domestic waste, trade effluent or farm waste, with or without it being diluted by surface water.

Traditionally foul or soil effluent is a discharge containing excreta; waste water is foul, but does not contain excreta or trade effluent.

Rain, surface, storm or ground water

This is natural water run off from the roof of buildings, paved areas, roads, car parks, etc., or ground water being that which is collected below ground by land drains or ditches. In its journey to the pipework systems it may become contaminated by 'soil' or chemicals, but not as a deliberate process.

Trade effluent

This is the fluid discharged from a manufacturing process or possibly a research or medical institute.

There is sometimes contention whether educational or health care buildings such as laboratories or laundries are manufacturing establishments. It is recommended that if in doubt an agreement should be made between the parties concerned and recorded in writing early in the design stage of a building as to the classification of the effluent and its treatment.

As previously indicated, it is the objective of the designer to provide the building or estate with pipework systems capable of conveying all the effluents discharged by all the attached equipment and sanitary ware to the satisfaction of the client and in accordance with the Statutory Rules and Regulations. He may also be required to provide a system for the removal of the rainwater falling on the building or estate, and to prevent flooding or dampness, which may necessitate a system of land drains. He may also be required to provide a system to protect the structure of the building by the removal of ground water.

Separate systems

The designer should provide a separate drainage system for the conveyance of the following:

(a) Foul or soil effluent.
(b) Rain, surface and ground water.
(c) Trade effluent.

The objective of segregating these three types of discharge is two-fold; firstly to present to the sewage or treatment works a regular flow of effluent of known quantity and content; and secondly, to prevent entry into the system anything which may knowingly damage the system or create a risk to the health of people.

Foul drainage

This system is provided to take away from the building any matter which cannot be disposed of to a water way or river without creating a risk to health. Once out of the building the effluent may be diluted with natural water (combined system) but usually links with a sewerage system for its ultimate treatment and disposal.

Rain, surface and ground water systems

This is a system provided to take only natural water from the roof of the buildings, paved areas, car parks and roads; it should not be contaminated with either foul or trade effluent.

It may be considered expensive to provide a double system from the roof of a multi-storey building (one pipe just to drain the roof and the other to serve the appliances), but it is infinitely preferable to the chaos that can prevail if a blockage develops at the wrong time.

Trade system (chemical drainage)

These two systems have been linked together because their effect on the drains, sewers and treatment works can be similar.

It is the mandatory duty of the building owner, and therefore delegated to the designer, not to allow the discharge of certain effluents into the sewerage system belonging to the authority responsible for the maintenance of the systems and the ultimate treatment of the effluent.

In general these prohibited effluents are (Public Health Act 1936):

(a) any matter likely to injure the sewer or drain or to interfere with the free flow of its contents or to effect prejudicially the treatment or disposal of its contents; or
(b) any chemical refuse or waste steam or any liquid of a temperature higher than 110 °F (43.3 °C) being refuse or steam which, or a liquid which when so heated is either alone or in combination with the contents of the sewer or drain dangerous, or the cause of a nuisance or prejudicial to health; or
(c) any petroleum spirit or carbide of calcium.

As the Act does not specify the quantities or concentrations of the chemicals that may be discharged it is the responsibility of the designer to discover from the client what is likely to be discharged and then to meet the representatives of the appropriate authority to agree the action to be taken.

Concentrated chemicals will require some treatment before being discharged into the main sewers, but dilute chemicals may be and are regularly discharged from the normal clean processes carried out by home occupiers.

Chemical systems

If it is agreed in discussions with the appropriate authority that dilution of the chemical effluent prior to discharge is acceptable, provision should be made for dilution holding tanks capable of taking a known quantity of chemical. More than one tank may be required and a method of switching the discharge from one tank to the other can be achieved with motorized penstock valves operated by float switches. A dousing mechanism may also be necessary to inject a neutralizing agent into the tanks.

Dilution should be carried out with water, but this need not be of potable quality. If conditions are suitable surface water stored on site can be economically used, but it is not possible to successfully dilute chemical effluent within the pipework system with rain water directly from roof surfaces.

In certain industrial estates with large roofs or car park areas it is possible to collect and store the surface water run off and use it for dilution. There is an added advantage in such a storage system which can also provide a static tank for fire fighting purposes. There must be, however, another source of dilution water in case of drought; bore holes, rivers or canals are all possibilities that the designer must investigate.

Chemical systems must be installed in suitable materials and the holding tanks must also be proof against attack which may cause leaking into the surrounding ground so that contamination of local ground water or chemical attack on adjacent structures does not occur.

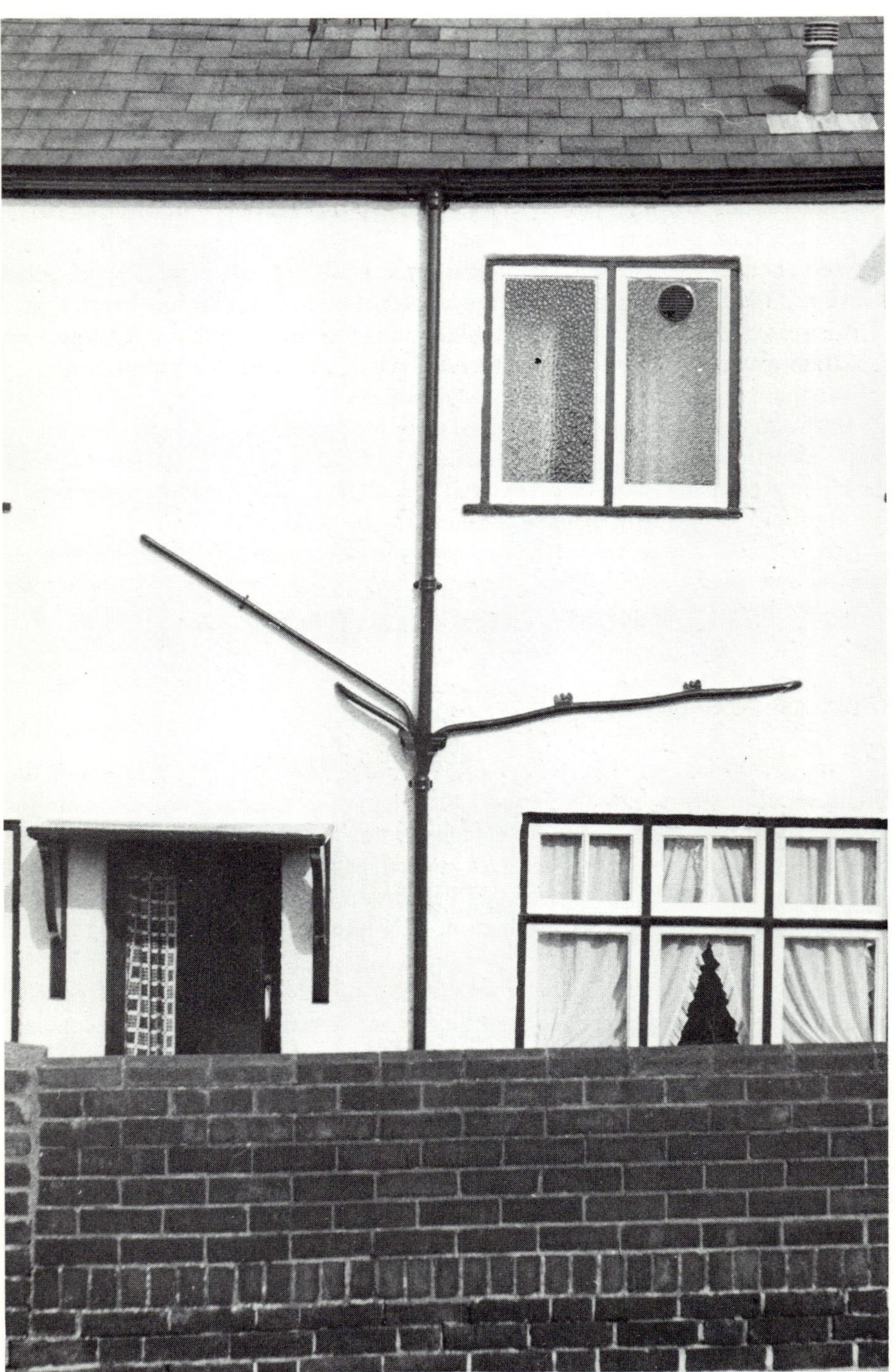

Fig. 3.1 Combined rainwater/waste system

Combined systems

These systems are often found in old buildings, where the roof water may discharge into the waste drainage system often attached to the face of the building.

The Building Regulations (N9.3 1976) are explicit in stating that no rainwater pipe shall be discharged into a soil or waste pipe unless the sewerage system is designed to cater for such a discharge, but the British Standard (BS 5572:1978), although discouraging the practice, recommends a limitation on the roof area of not more than 40 m^2 that may be drained into a discharge stack, and the height of the building to be not more than ten storeys.

It is recommended that for any building the rainwater and foul discharges are separated except for very small areas such as balconies, etc. If the balcony trap

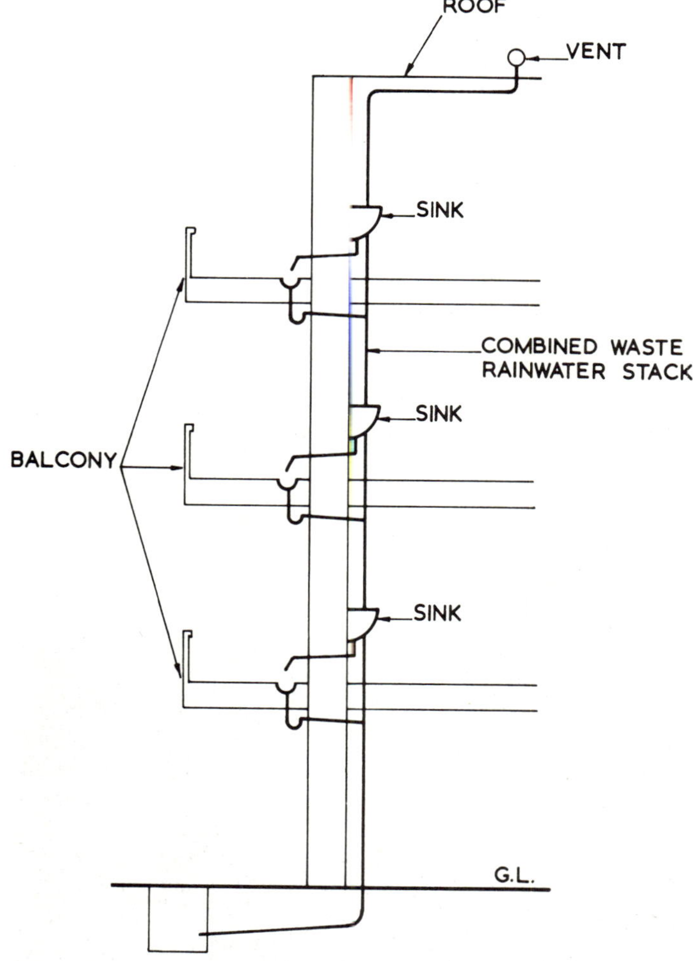

Fig. 3.2 Balcony drains to foul system

was to dry out it would become an open vent for the foul drain; provision should therefore be made to top up this trap.

Above-ground foul systems

This is a system of pipework collecting the discharges from those appliances situated on all floors (except the ground floor) including an undercroft.

Traditionally these discharges were separated into 'soil' and 'waste' and the Building Regulations 1976 still identifies soil and waste appliances and soil and waste pipes, although the British Standard 5572 only lists 'discharge pipes', conveying the discharge from sanitary appliances.

As all the effluent (except chemical or trade effluents) from all the appliances ends up in the same underground drain the designer need not be too interested

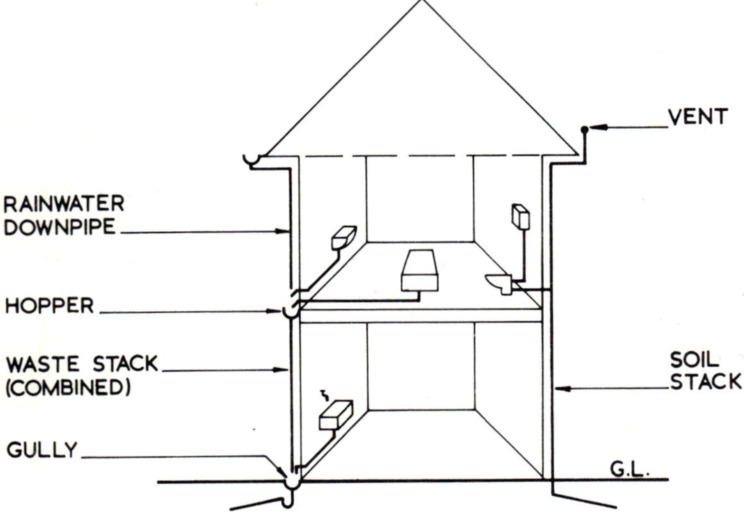

Fig. 3.3 Typical traditional domestic system

in the differentiations between the terms soil and waste. Many traditional dwellings have separate soil and waste systems on the external face of the building and the 1976 Regulations allow a soil or waste pipe to be placed outside the external wall of a building having not more than three storeys except that the waste pipe shall not discharge into a hopper head.

For many years prior to the 1976 Regulations all new dwellings had to have their discharge stacks contained within the building to prevent damage by freezing.

Over the years various names have been given to the types of vertical discharge systems in vogue at the time; these have been rationalized into four basic

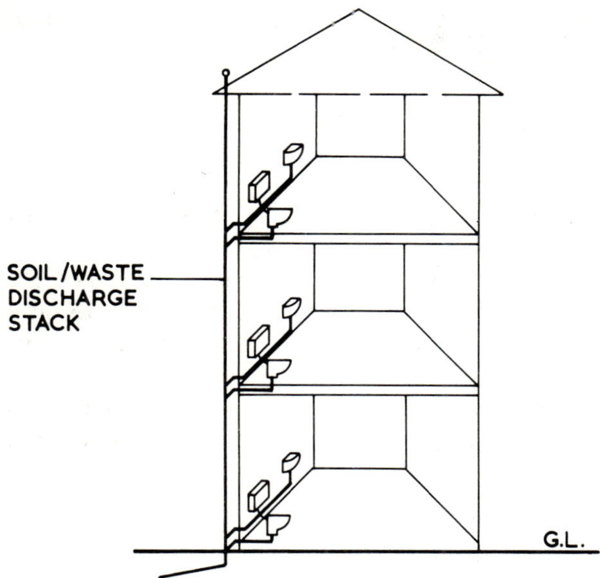

Fig. 3.4 External soil/waste (discharge) stack for up to three storeys

systems suitable, with some modifications, for all types of buildings and covered by BS 5572.

In all these cases the single appliance shown in the figures connected to a discharge pipe may be replaced by more than one appliance.

(a) Single stack system.
(b) Modified single stack system.
(c) Ventilated system.
(d) Horizontal system (not specifically covered by BS 5572).

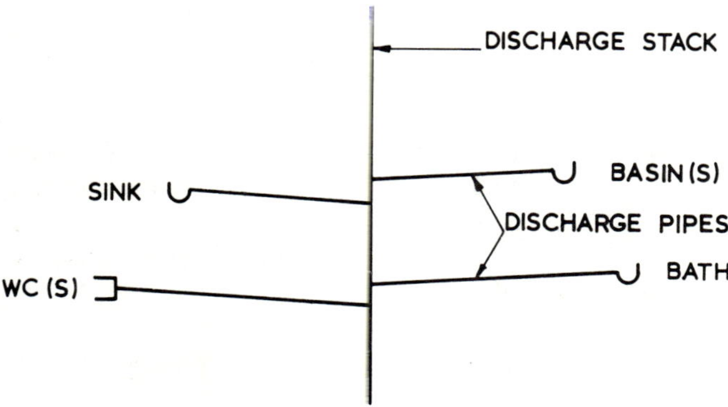

Fig. 3.5 Single stack system

Single stack system

This uses, at it implies, one stack to take all the discharges from appliances. The stack must be large enough to control the pressure fluctuations that will occur within the stack.

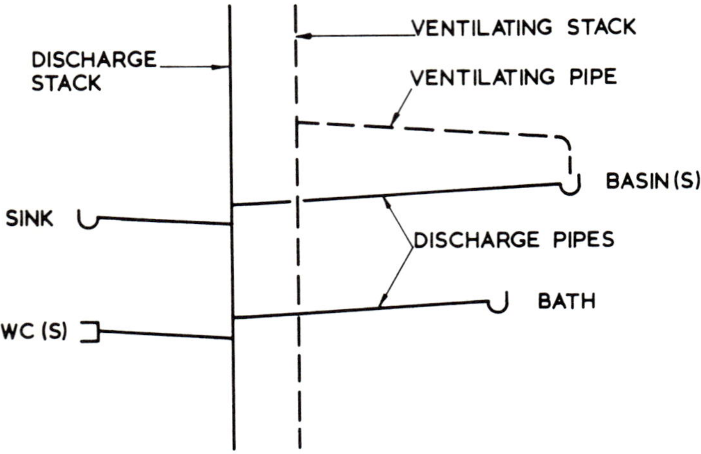

Fig. 3.6 Modified single stack system

Modified single stack system

This method incorporates an end vent either directly to atmosphere, to a vent stack or fitted with an air admittance valve. It can be used when the limitations of the single stack system are exceeded.

Ventilated stack system

This can be used in situations where close grouping of appliances creates pressure fluctuations that must be alleviated by the additional ventilation of the single stack.

Ventilated system

This is where every appliance or group of appliances has individual vent connections.

It is traditional in application, expensive in labour and material and should only be used when all other design techniques have been researched.

Whatever system of internal discharge pipework is provided it is important that it must be so designed that the installation is reasonably accessible for maintenance and repair throughout its entire length.

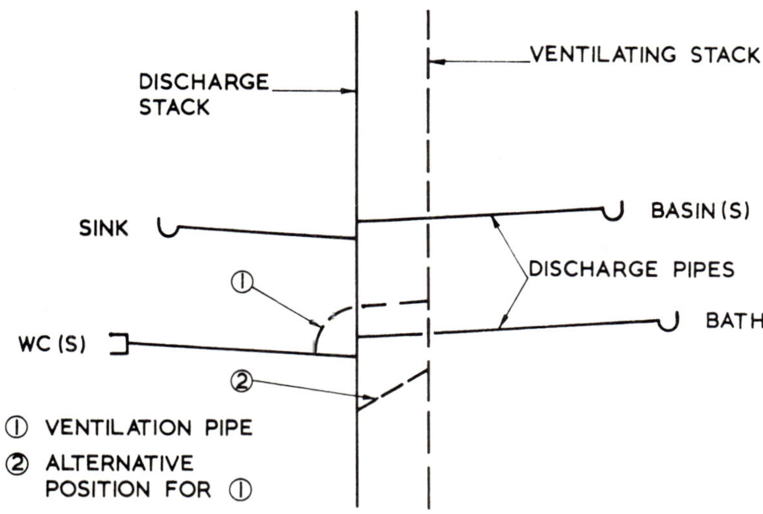

Fig. 3.7 Ventilated stack system

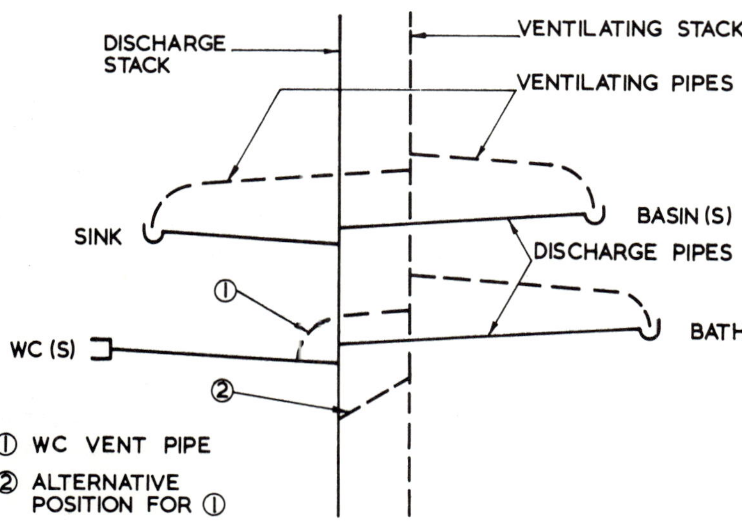

Fig. 3.8 Ventilated system

Horizontal systems

These may have to be used where the vertical penetration of the building structure is not acceptable to the client. These structures must therefore have deep inter-floor/ceiling voids for all services and full co-ordination will be necessary to avoid clashes.

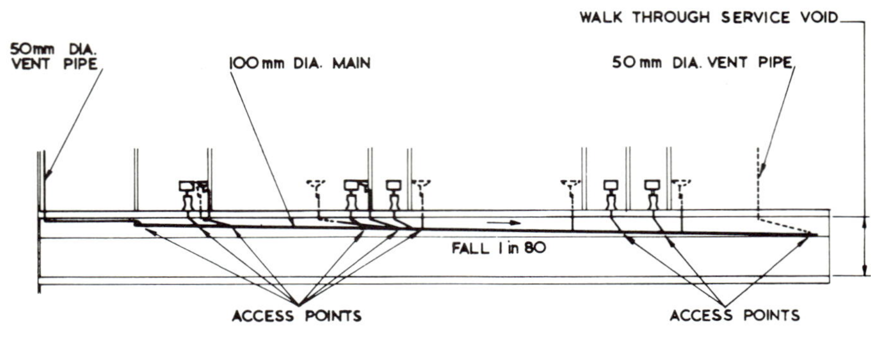

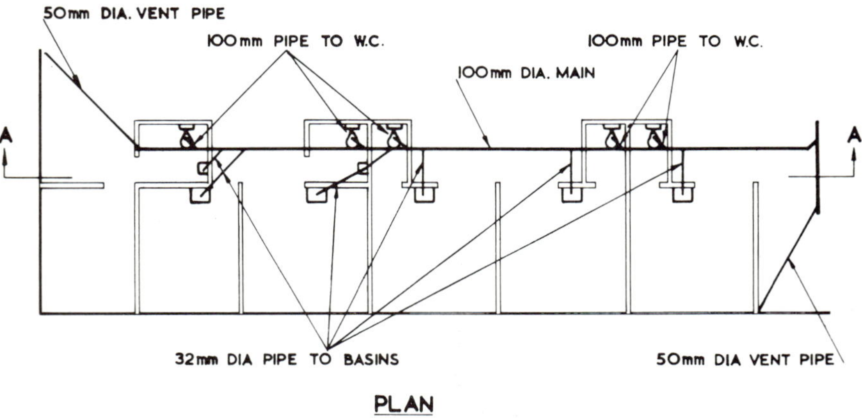

Fig. 3.9 Horizontal system; Grenwich District Hospital

Venting will be required, usually at the ends of main runs, and air admittance valves may be used to allow air into the system.

Above-ground rainwater systems

The design of the rainwater drainage system for any roof structure will depend upon the profile of the roof of which there are two basic types: pitched and flat.

Pitched roof drainage

In its most basic form this type of roof will have gutters fixed at the eaves of the pitch, but they may be external to the roof structure (Fig. 3.10b) or internal (Fig. 3.10a). The down pipes may also be external or internal, when the design requirements are for of performance standards which must comply with the regulations for discharge pipes.

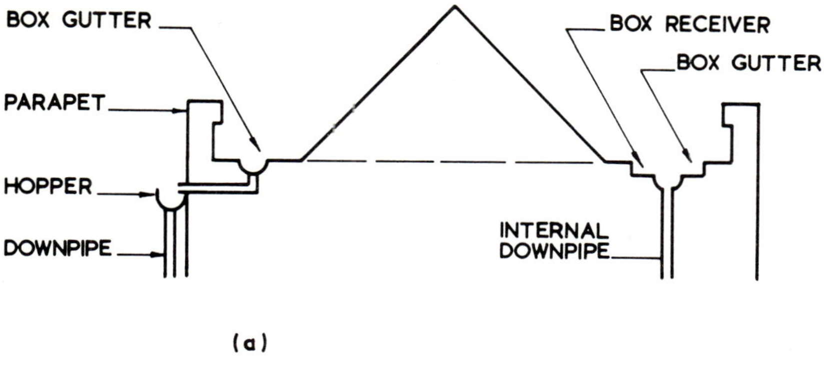

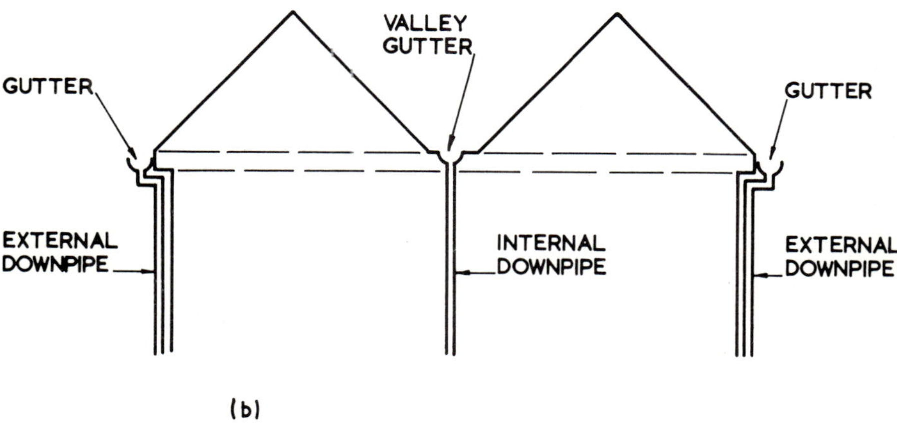

Fig. 3.10 Types of pitched roof rainwater systems

Pitched roofs may be added together (Fig. 3.10b); this form of roof is often used as a lightweight construction for large-plan factories. The junctions between the pitches forms valleys in which a valley gutter must be provided. It is very important that this gutter is correctly sized and installed, as failure will mean water overflowing into the building.

Provision must be made to allow the valley gutter to overflow external to the building – usually by a wear overflow at the end (in case a blockage of the downpipe or outlet occurs), and it is advisable to provide slatted walk boards down the length of the gutter to prevent both damage to the material of the gutter by maintenance operatives and to hold snow so that it may drip through on thawing and not block the gutter or outlets.

Flat roof drainage

The use of the word 'flat' is a misnomer as it usually refers to a roof whose outer surface is nearly horizontal or inclined at an angle not exceeding 10 degrees.

Eaves gutters can be used for flat roofs and the design rules are then similar to those for pitched roof systems of drainage, but often flat roofs are finished with parapets or upstands of some form and the roof must be drained by a system of outlets integrated with the pitch plan of the area.

It is always advisable to position some of the outlets at the corners and periphery of the building and the designer must bear in mind that as all buildings settle – possibly unevenly – it is inadvisable to rely on outlets positioned only on pitch junctions down the centre line of a roof. Too often the drainage of a flat roof is left to chance, the designer providing sufficient outlets in the hope that the water will find its way to them.

It is recommended that the provision of box gutters at parapets and longitudinal box gutters across the roof will provide a good drainage system.

If not released foul air will occur next to windows or ventilation systems. It is not necessary to provide flat roof outlets with traps, which would require planned maintenance.

Blockages

The problem of rainwater gutters and down pipes becoming blocked is not so acute as with discharge pipes, but it is just as important, as rainwater overflowing within a building can cause damage to the fabric and structure. The resulting general dampness may also affect the health of the occupants.

Blockages are caused by objects preventing the free flow of the water into and/or within the gutters, outlets or down pipes. Leaves and paper may block gutters, gullies and down pipes and balls have also been known to lodge in outlets.

If leaves or needles from trees are likely to enter the system seasonal planned maintenance must be undertaken. An annual inspection should also be carried out to ascertain the condition of the system and a procedure organized to deal with emergencies.

Below-ground foul drainage

This system can be sub-divided into two parts – that which collects the discharges from appliances on the ground floor and may be internal to the building, and the drainage external to the building or buildings and usually carrying the collected effluent to the treatment works or the authority sewerage system.

Internal below-ground drainage

The mandatory rules for pipework systems buried in the ground are different

Fig. 3.11 (facing page) Flat roof box gutters

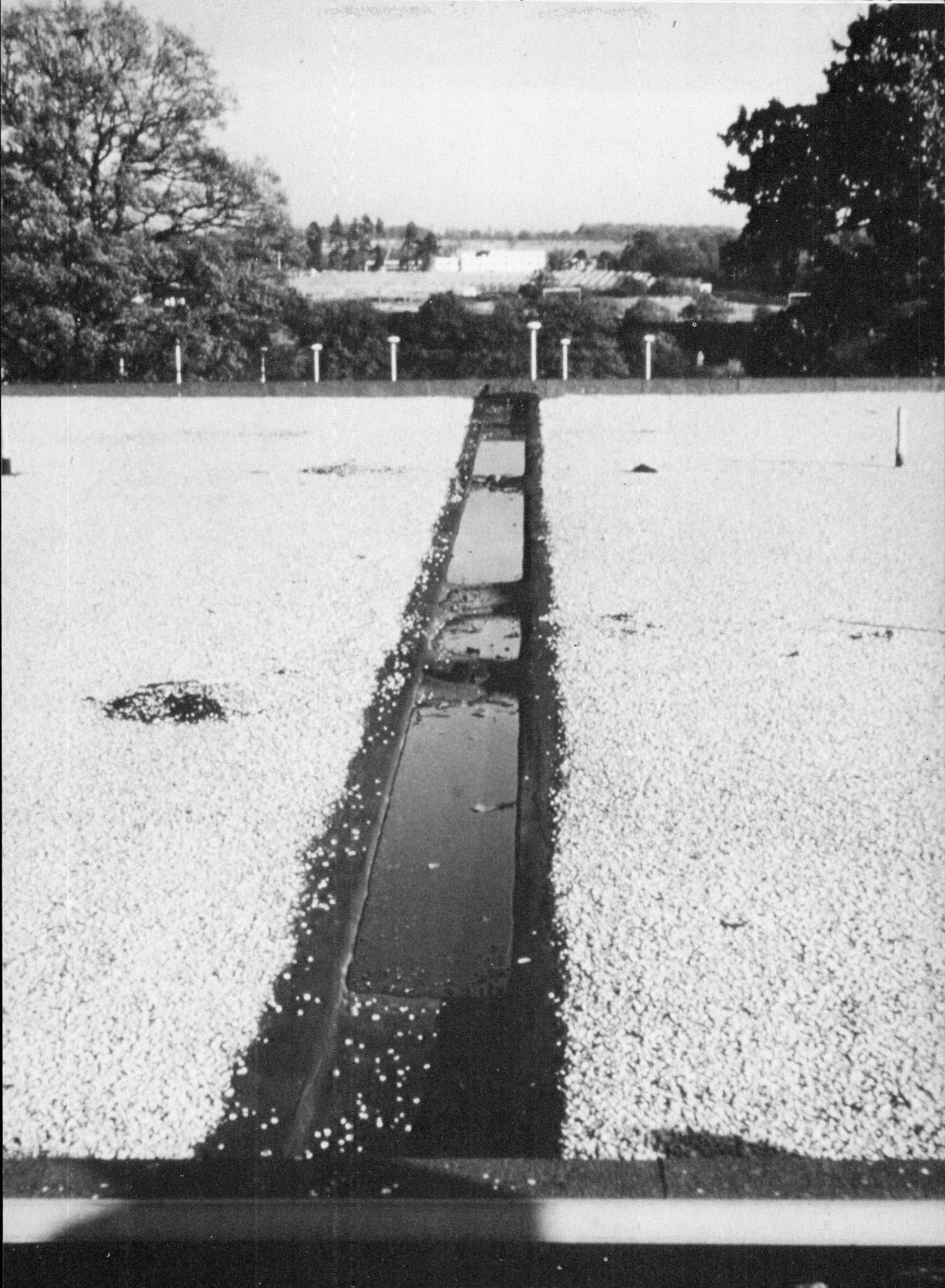

from those for horizontal systems, either above the ground or in undercrofts. The smallest diameter pipe allowed in an underground situation is 75 mm, so that a single basin fitted with a spray tap on a solid ground floor has to discharge into a 75 mm drain; but in all other cases it may discharge into a 32 mm waste.

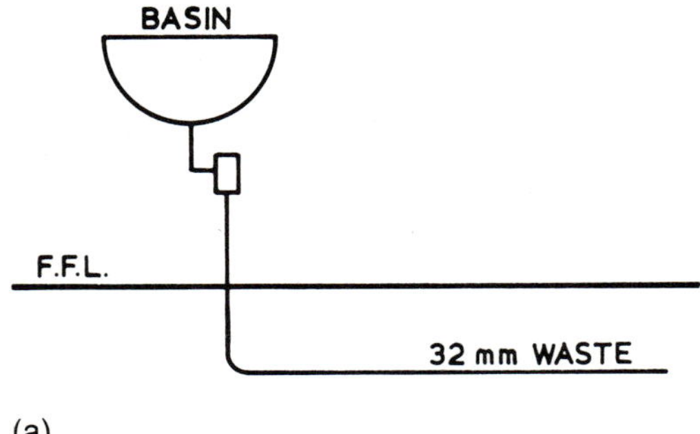

(a)

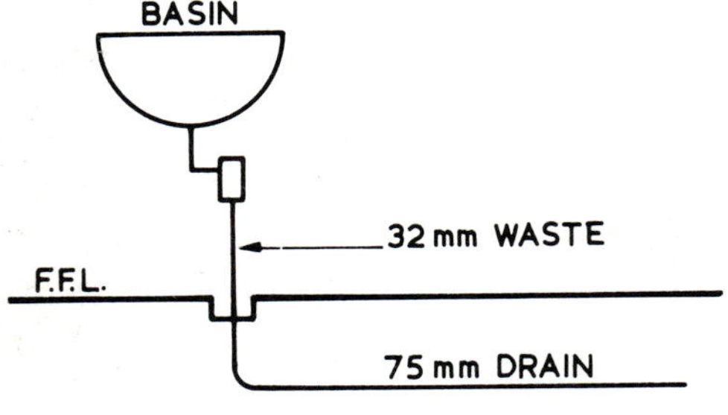

(b)

Fig. 3.12 Basin waste/drain
(a) Undercroft/Above ground floor drainage situation
(b) Ground floor drainage situation

All other underground drains must have an internal diameter of not less than 100 mm if they carry soil water or trade effluent, and all systems must have such means of access as may be necessary for inspection and maintenance, which means the provision of rodding points, manholes and inspection chambers.

The position of internal manholes must be carefully considered by the designer before he plans his main drainage runs as they must be quickly and easily accessible for the purpose for which they were intended, i.e. maintenance. They should not be sited where maintenance will impede the free movement of persons or goods, or where stores may be stacked on top of them.

The covers should be pressure tight to prevent sewage leaking out of the chamber in the event of a blockage down stream.

It is recommended that only sealed drainage systems are used internally, and in critical areas such as food preparation or chemical zones blockage indicators should be fitted in the chambers.

External below-ground drainage

The design of foul underground drainage external to the building should follow the same rules as that of the internal system. Fewer manholes will be required as there are likely to be fewer branch connections; consequently fewer blockages may be experienced due to the greater and more continuous flow within the system.

The positioning of access points and manholes must again be carefully considered; they should not be positioned in roads or car parks, or in any position where they may become inaccessible either due to obstructions, traffic movement or hidden by landscaping or detritus.

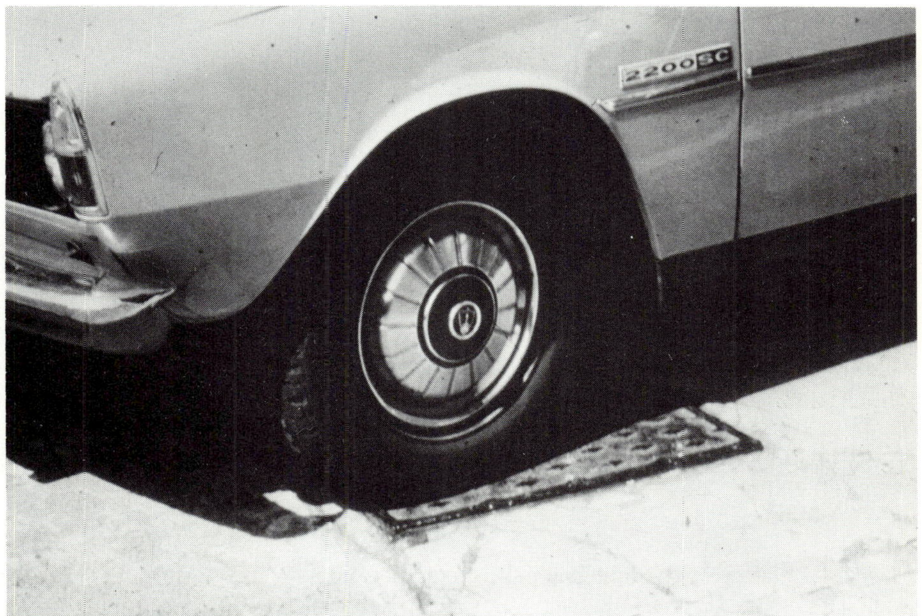

Fig. 3.13 Manhole blocked by car

When developing the outline plan of an external drainage system for an estate or large building project it is essential that the designer becomes involved with the positioning of buildings on the site so that the most economical drainage system can be considered. At some time he must provide a main outfall into the authority sewerage system and he should take account of the natural ground contours.

It is inadvisable to develop the internal and periphery systems before considering the final outfall positions in relation to all the ground factors.

The mechanical engineer must be kept informed of the underground drainage network and consultation may be necessary to prevent the clashing of services. It is not unknown for an underground service duct required by the mechanical engineer from the boiler house to the building to effectively block the route to the main drain outfall from the building to the authority sewer, thereby dropping the inverts and requiring pumping to be included in the development.

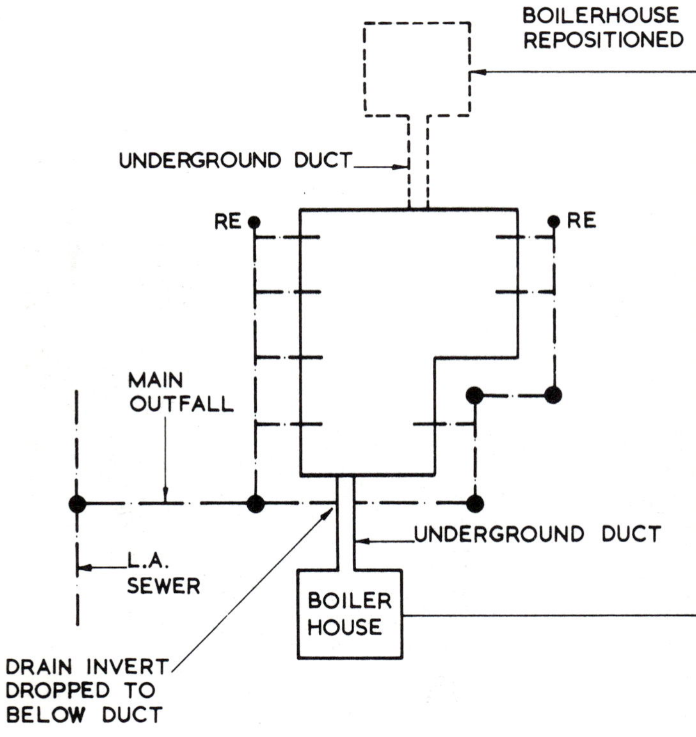

Fig. 3.14 Problems of co-ordinating underground services

Below-ground rain and surface water drainage

The rainwater down pipes from the roof of any building must be connected into the drainage system in a similar manner as the foul discharge stacks. By the careful planning of inverts it may be possible to contain both the underground surface water and foul drains into one trench with a consequent considerable

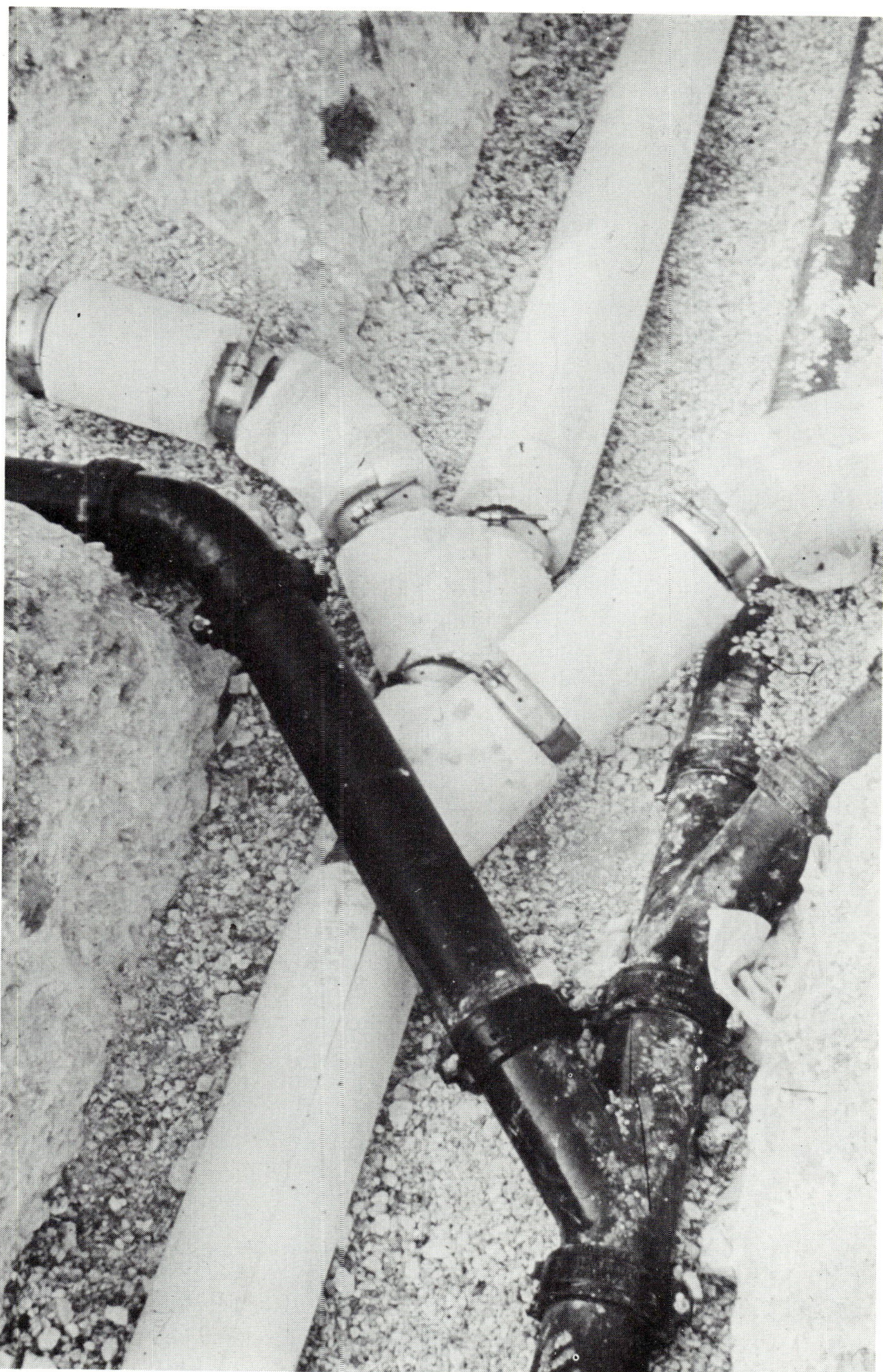

Fig. 3.15 Spun iron and glass drains sharing same trench

saving in the cost of excavation and backfilling and ground reinstatement. This system necessitates manholes large enough to contain two 100 mm or 150 mm pipes; the soil or foul drain must always be a sealed system to prevent overflow into the surface water drain, which may be an open channel.

It will therefore not be necessary to provide a standing plug as required in a single pipe sealed system to drain water from the manhole.

Soakaways

The use of soakaways to take all or some of the surface water run-off from an estate may only be considered if the ground is suitable for its dispersal.

The rate water disperses into the ground will depend upon the permeability of the soil which will vary from place to place.

All clays such as London, Oxford and Gault are almost impervious and the use of soakaways should not be considered, but sands and gravels can be very permeable and soakaways then can be used with confidence. Between these two soil types is a whole range with varying permeabilities.

Chalk soils should be carefully examined for swallow holes and these may form into soakaways and any constructed should be sited well away from the building or structure to avoid the possibility of collapse.

If the designer doubts the permeability of the soil he should initiate tests to discover the rate at which water will disperse. These tests should also show the possible ground water table and should be carried out in wet conditions, preferably in the month with the highest local rainfall.

Bore holes should be taken down to a depth of 1 m, and if a 150 mm auger is used and 300 mm depth of water added it will equal 5½ litres. The time of dispersal should be recorded and the test repeated so that the effect of possible waterlogging can be noted. The bore hole should then be taken down in 1 m drops and the tests repeated until the actual soakaway depth has been reached. The rate of dispersal can then be quantified against the run-off rate from the area to be drained and the size and depth of the soakaway calculated.

Soakaways may be constructed in two forms – filled and unfilled – but it is recommended that filled forms are only used for the drainage of very small surface areas in soils of high permeability as they are likely to become choked; their effectiveness will, in time, be reduced.

Unfilled soakaways are similar in construction to manholes with side walls that allow the water out.

Combined drainage

In certain parts of the country, and particularly in old inner city areas, it is pointless and unnecessary to provide separate systems between the building periphery drains and the sewer outfall as the authority sewer will inevitably be 'combined'. In this case the two drains, foul and surface water, can be joined

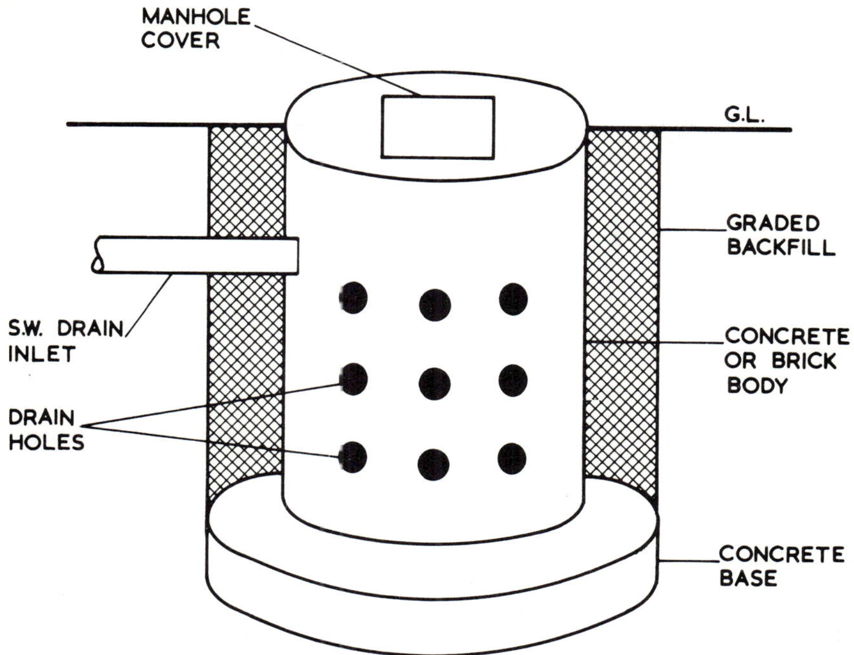

Fig. 3.16 Typical soakaway

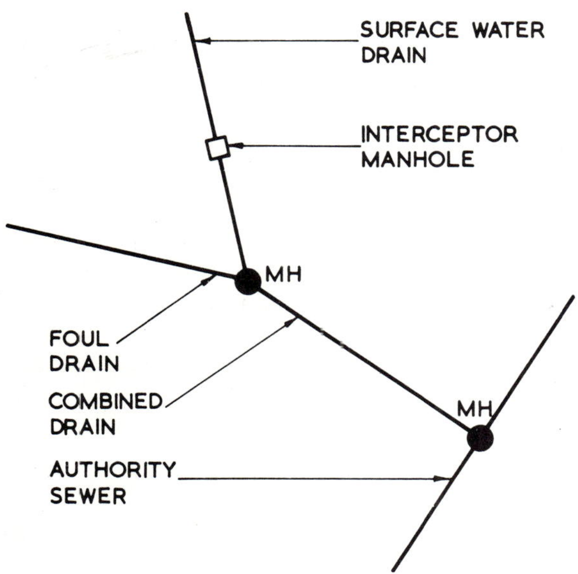

Fig. 3.17 Combined surface water and foul drainage

together at some convenient manhole, and to prevent foul sewer gasses venting via untrapped rain or surface water outlets an interceptor must be provided.

Under no circumstances should an interceptor be provided on the foul system as they are not required under any statutory regulation and are well known as a main cause of drain blockages.

Surface and rainwater gullies

In certain circumstances the collection of surface water must be undertaken by gullies, particularly from paved areas and car parks, etc., although the use of channels is to be preferred.

It is unnecessary to discharge rainwater stacks or down pipes into or over gullies as it is constructionally expensive and provides points requiring planned maintenance. A direct connection with an associated rodding point is to be preferred (Figs. 12.14 and 12.15).

Land drains

Ground water – water underground, either static or moving, is often found when developing virgin sites in rural areas. Local knowledge, names and large-scale Ordnance Survey maps may assist the designer in ascertaining the possibility of ground water, and such names as 'Spring Meadow' or 'Water Meadow' and the growth of rushes or willow trees will advertise the possible presence of water.

The redevelopment of existing sites may also necessitate the provision of land drains to pick up existing systems, divert ground water movement or improve grassed areas.

A new building often interrupts the natural flow of ground water – or breaks through an existing land drainage system that may have been installed for agricultural purposes.

If the foundations of the building go below the water table provision must be made to divert the water away from the foundations.

It may also be necessary to provide land drains to landscaped areas or grassed areas used for recreational purposes. They will also be required at the base of embankments to prevent water running off on to road surfaces; motorways in particular have elaborate land drains along all sides to assist in keeping the surfaces free from water.

Land drains should always be provided with a rodding eye at the top end to enable the system to be cleaned out at planned intervals.

If a land drain discharges into either a surface water or combined drain a mud sump must be provided to prevent sedimentation entering the system. This mud sump will require planned maintenance.

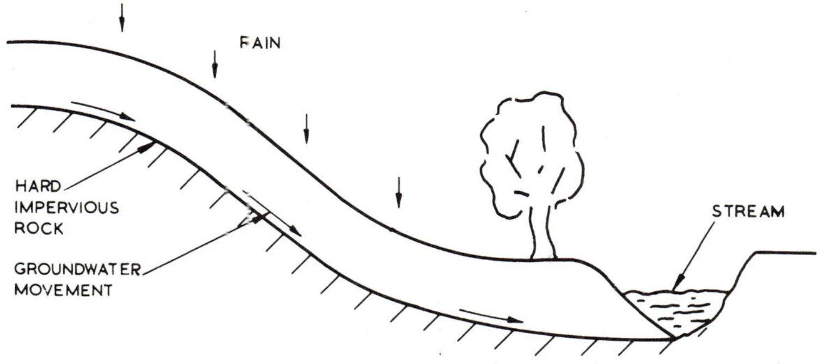

a. CROSS SECTION OF SITE

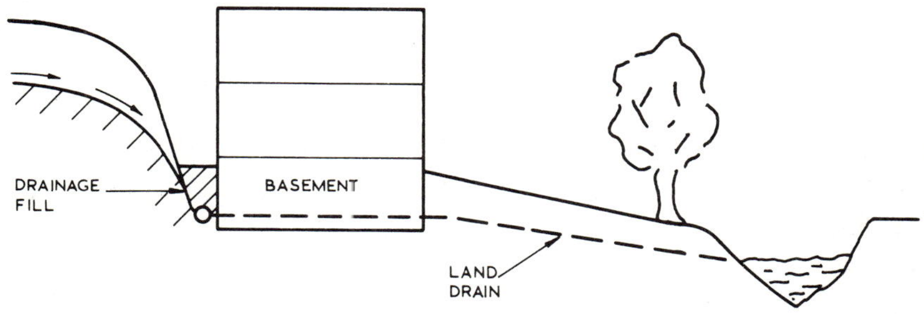

b. CROSS SECTION OF BUILDING ON SITE

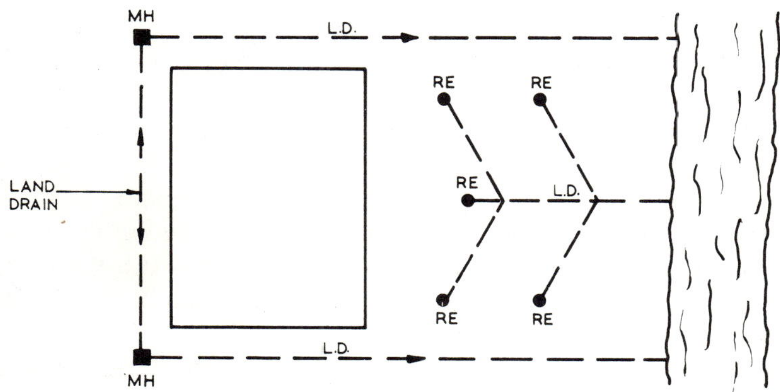

c. PLAN SHOWING LAND DRAINS AND MAINTENANCE POINTS

Fig. 3.18 Land drainage

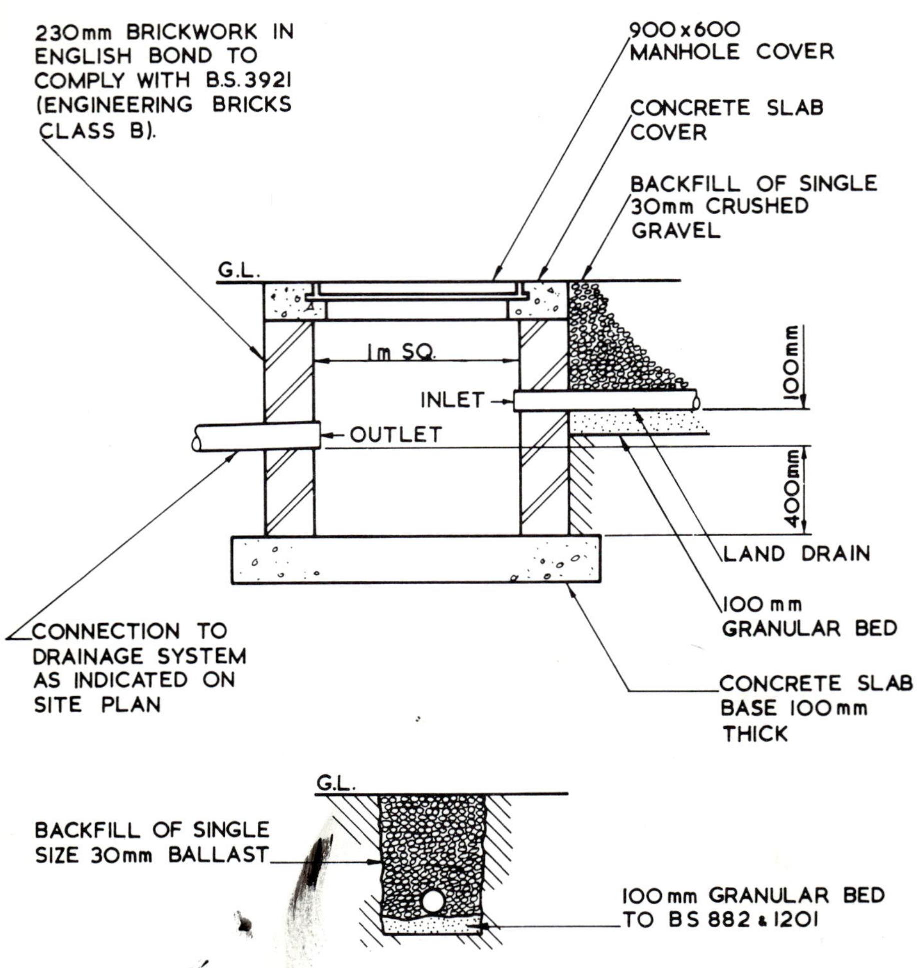

Fig. 3.19 Typical mud sump

Drainage to water courses

Rather than provide an elaborate system of surface water drains it may often be possible to discharge into ditches, streams or rivers. This will usually entail obtaining the permission of the appropriate river authority and may necessitate obtaining a right of way across adjacent land.

The construction of the outfall is important so that erosion of the bank opposite does not occur. Protection to the end of the outfall must be provided to prevent children or animals entering the pipe, particularly when it is not flowing.

It is not advisable to have the outfall below average river level and a tidal flap valve should be fitted to prevent debris floating up into the outfall drain when the river rises.

Chapter 4

Systems materials (pipes and fittings)

Introduction

The choice of materials for any drainage system must be taken with due regard to a number of important influencing factors.

1. Its suitability for the effluents that are likely to be carried over the life of the systems at their concentrations and temperatures.
2. Safety.
3. That it meets the design requirements in terms of flow capacity; it is manufactured in the required sizes.
4. It is structurally and mechanically stable for the particular application.
5. Is it likely to block?
6. Is it readily available in all the sizes and fittings required?
7. As installed, including any support system required, is it cost competitive with the alternative materials?

All the above factors influence the designer's choice, but the installation, timing and availability of both materials and specialist labour must also be taken into account.

For overseas work the designer must also consider that skilled labour may not be available and therefore any pipework system that can be easily assembled by a jointing system capable of being taught to local labour is attractive. The availability of materials must also be considered – it is not always possible to telephone a local stockist for the 'rep.' to bring a missing fitting to the site the following day when the site is in the Arabian desert. The vulnerability of the material must therefore also be taken into account; breakages can hold up a contract.

Suitability

Most domestic type effluents are innocuous to pipework materials and, except for high temperature and chemically charged discharges, can be carried by all the materials listed.

It is in the design of laboratory and industrial process plant drainage systems where chemical effluents are likely, and also in industrial kitchens and food preparation establishments where long periods of very high temperature discharges may be experienced, that the choice of systems materials becomes more complex.

It must be remembered that once a building is in use the client will not welcome the inconvenience caused by 'adjusting' the system, e.g. changing materials: it is extremely expensive to replace a failed underground drain, particularly when it is under the building. Claims for damages against the designer by a client will not enhance his reputation.

Although many 'plastics' – except unplasticized PVC and MPVC – will take intermittent discharges of very high temperature effluents, particularly in above ground or undercroft situations, these materials are subject to considerable differential thermal movement and if not corrrectly fixed – in some cases by a continuous support system – they will snake between fixings.

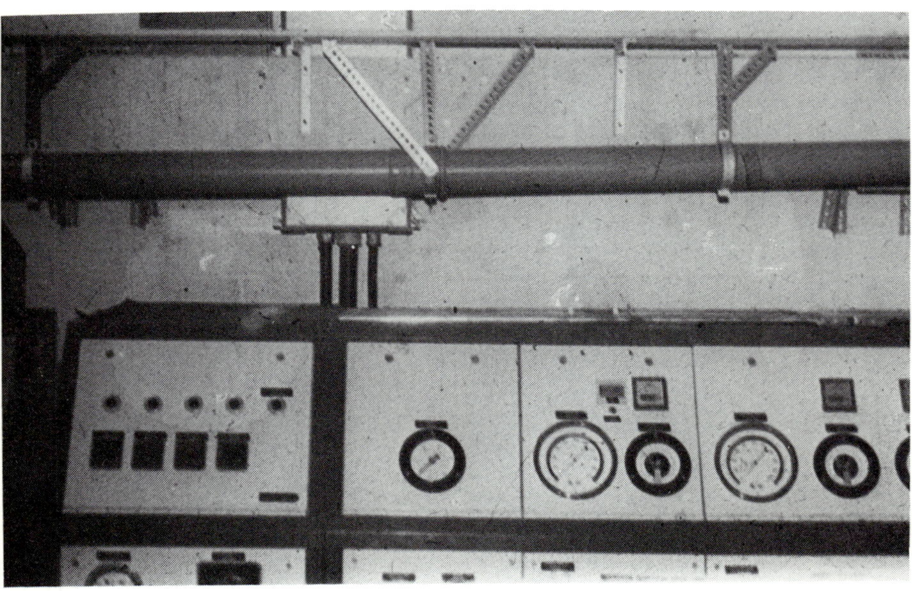

Fig. 4.1 Manufacturers support test rig for unplasticized PVC pipe

In an underground situation the heat from the effluent is absorbed into the walls of the pipework and cannot be readily dissipated into the surrounding fill which acts like an insulating blanket (in above ground situations it is dissipated by convection into the surrounding air), consequently the pipe may soften and deform or collapse. There is therefore no advantage for the designer in specifying plastic systems for the conveyance of very high temperature intermittent or high temperature continuous discharges, although he may be tempted to do so when the effluents are chemically charged.

Laboratories, including hospital pathology departments, usually do not discharge large quantities of either high temperature or concentrated chemical effluents, but it does happen – particularly in teaching laboratories – that an accidental breakage of a container may occur and the contents flushed into the pipework system with possible disastrous consequences to the material.

In industrial process plants the management is only interested in production – not drainage, and the type, concentration and temperature of the effluent may change with the manufacturing process. Often very large quantities of chemically charged effluents, sometimes at high temperatures, are discharged through the drainage system to treatment or recovery plants. As the designer will therefore be unsure of the effluent likely to be discharged over even a few years he must 'play safe' and only specify a material that can carry 99 per cent of all commercial chemicals likely to be used and at a varying temperature range. The only material known to the author that meets this specification is borosilicate glass (see p. 51).

Safety

This may appear to be an unusual requirement related to drainage materials, but under certain circumstances inappropriate pipework material may create a health hazard by leaking, breaking or exploding, thereby endangering persons maintaining or working the vicinity of the system.

Certain pipework systems, because of the properties of the material, may soften or leak at the joints, or corrode through, and leak small quantities of possibly pathogenic, radioactive or chemical effluent into ducts or ceiling voids where it could be potentially dangerous to either people or the fabric of the building.

Chemicals such as azide solutions when in contact with metal pipes combine to form percussive compounds of metallic azides and a system so contaminated may explode if impacted. This is a likely effect during maintenance.

Flow

When designing a total pipework system including the selection of the fittings the sizes available can be a controlling factor.

The choice of size can affect layout and is dictated by the anticipated maximum hydraulic load (flow) and the carrying capacity of the system related to available gradients without pumping, all of which must be considered.

The sizes required to meet the maximum anticipated peak flow must be checked with the manufacturer or at least his up-to-date literature.

In certain circumstances, particularly when designing chemical systems, double or even triple banking may be necessary due to the maximum manufactured size of a material that must be specified.

Stability

The structural and mechanical stability of a material is usually only an influ-

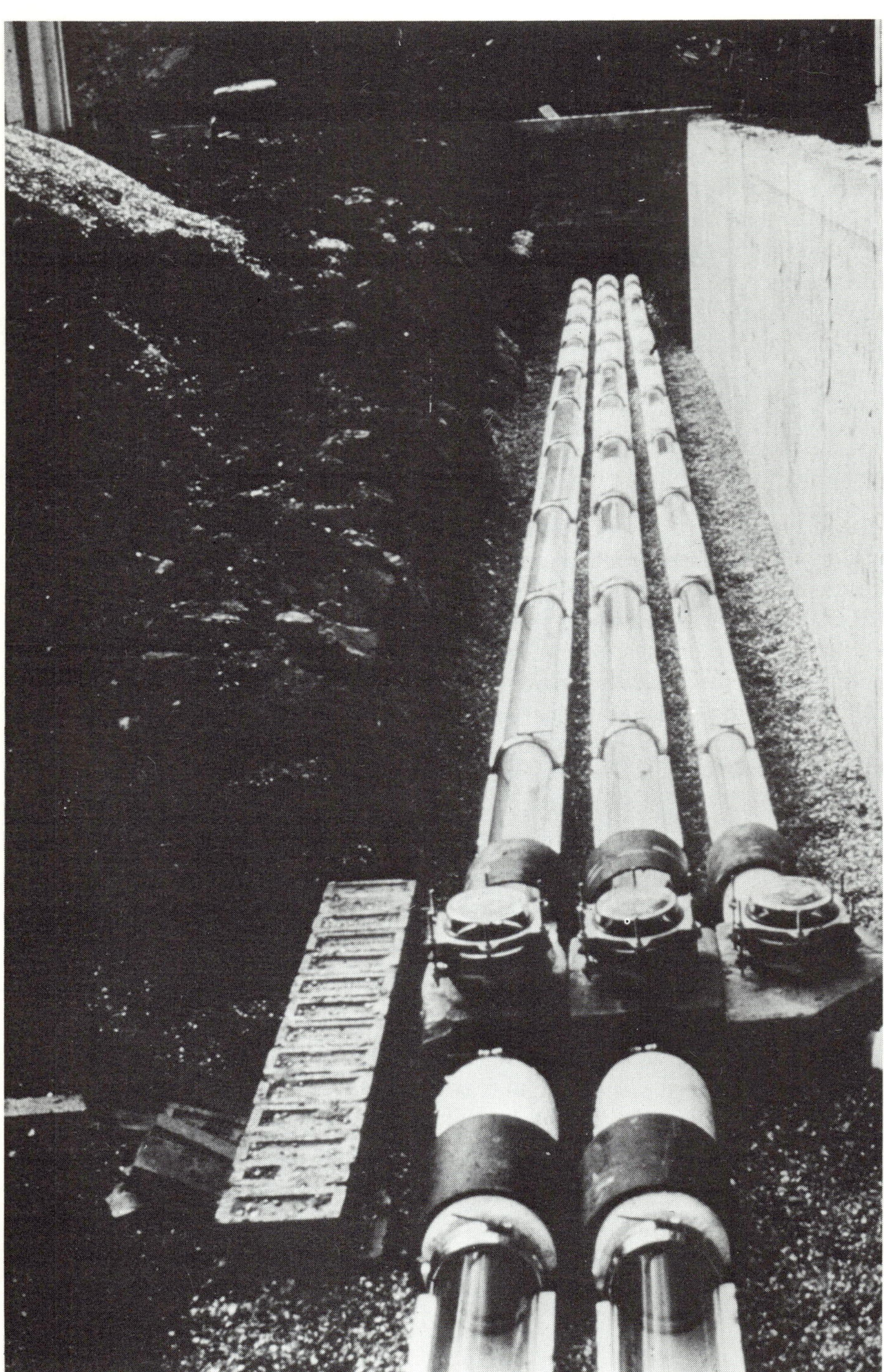

Fig. 4.2 Banking of glass system underground

encing factor in material selection when it is likely to be either exposed to mechanical damage or used underground.

In certain circumstances external down pipes may be liable to physical damage and should therefore be installed for at least 2 m above ground in a structurally strong material such as iron.

Soils that are liable to movement such as loose sand or made up ground will offer little support to the walls of buried pipes, with the consequence that plastic or pitch fibre systems may be deformed by the superimposed load of the ground above. Where pipework is installed underground, but near the surface or adjacent to the passage of heavy traffic, pipework should be structurally strong, but flexible.

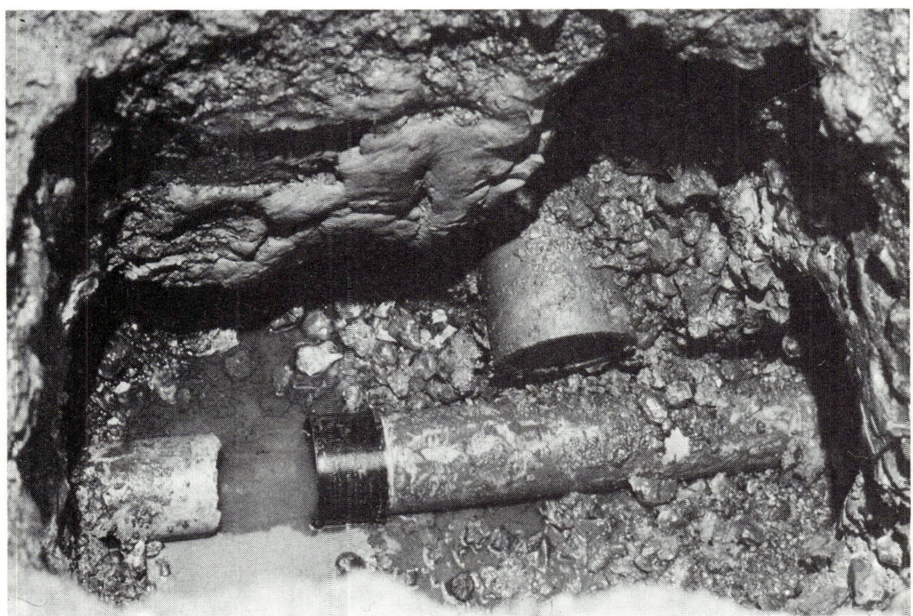

Fig. 4.3 Broken underground clay drain

Blockages

Blockages will occur in any pipework system that is of rough bore, with crudely made fittings and a jointing system between components that does not accurately align the spigot and socket, or where the system is easily deformed or broken by mechanical means. Gradients do not influence the likelihood of blockages developing as much as the quality of the material and the installation.

Costs

The cost competitiveness of any drainage system can be divided between the cost of materials, pipes and fittings, and the cost of installation.

For above-ground systems this will include the fixing system, and underground the cost of excavation, bedding and backfilling of the trench.

When examining the total cost of any drainage system for an above-ground installation the added cost of the fire officer's requirements must also be taken into account. Most plastics, except PVC, are flammable, they will burn and continue to burn once ignited, as will pitch fibre. The cost of providing fire ducts may therefore influence the choice of materials.

Materials

The following materials are used for the manufacture of drainage pipes and fittings, either for above- or below-ground installation, or in some cases both situations.

This list is not intended to be a catalogue of materials, as most of them are adequately covered by a British Standard Specification, but it is intended to draw to the designer's attention some of their advantages and disadvantages from a user's point of view.

Plastics

There are a number of plastics used for drainage purposes, usually qoted by their initials as follows:

ABS Acrylonitrile Butadine Styrene.
HDPE High Density Polyethylene.
PP Polypropylene.
UPVC Unplasticized Polyvinyl Chloride.
MPVC Modified UPVC.
GRP Glass-reinforced plastics.

Pipes and fittings manufactured in ABS, HDPE and PP are usually of small diameter and often used for waste systems.

They are resistant to many dilute chemicals particularly those used in domestic buildings and capable of conveying intermittent discharges of high temperature effluents such as produced by washing machines and dishwashers.

Acrylonitrile batadene styrene and PVC systems can be solvent welded, but HDPE and PP in domestic systems are connected together by mechanical or push fit connectors.

PP components can also be joined together by fusion welding, often successfully used for laboratory drainage systems and available for commercial systems in sizes up to 100 mm diameter. It is, however, adversely affected by a number of chemicals and prior to its specification the designer should verify the composition of the effluents to be discharged over the life of the system (Table 4.2).

All plastic systems are very versatile when used with mechanical couplings or

Table 4.1 Chemicals that will adversely affect polypropylene. Classification C should be adequate for intermittent contact if diluted. Class D chemicals must not enter the system without some damage being accepted.
(The higher the temperature the greater the reaction.)

	Temperature	
	20 °C	*60 °C*
Amyl acetate	—	C
Amyl chloride	C	C
Benzene	—	C
Bromine liquid	D	—
Bromine water	C	—
Butyl acetate	—	C
Carbon disulphide	—	C
Carbon tetrachloride	C	C
Chlorine gas	D	D
Chlorine gas, wet	—	D
Chlorobenzene	C	C
Chloroform	C	D
Chlorosulphonic acid	D	D
Chromic/sulphuric acid	D	D
Cyclohexanone	—	C
Decalin	C	C
Ethyl chloride	C	C
Furfural	C	C
Gasoline	—	C
Gas liquor	C	—
Iso-octane	C	C
Methylethylketone	—	C
Methylene chloride	C	—
Nitric acid 90% aq. sol	D	D
Nitric acid 70% aq. sol	C	D
Nitric acid 50% aq. sol	—	D
50–50 HNO_3–HCl	—	D
Oleum	D	D
Petrol	—	C
Petroleum ether (BP 100–140 °C)	C	C
Sulphuric acid	C	C
50–50 H_2SO_4/HNO_3	C	D
Tetrahydrofuran	C	C
Tetralin	C	C
Toluene	C	C
Transformer oil	—	C
Trichloroethylene	C	C
Turpentine	C	C
White spirit	—	C
Xylene	C	C

'0' ring joints that can easily be broken down and remade again, but the fusion welding technique requires the use of special heating equipment. Skill is necessary in making fusion joints and some practice is required to get the 'feel' of the process. It is important that the joint being made is allowed to get up to temperature and not hurried or subjected to cold draughts. If improperly made the system can fail under test, or in operation over a period of time due to the effect of the considerable differential thermal movement inherent to this material.

Correctly made fusion welded joints become a homogenous continuous length – the joint ceases to exist – and becomes a length of pipe with a double thickness over the socket.

Table 4.2 Coefficients of thermal expansion and relevant temperatures for drainage materials

Material	*Expansion coefficient*		*Softening point*	
ABS	7	11×10^{-5}	93	105 °C
HDPE	12	16×10^{-5}	110	130 °C
PP	11	17×10^{-5}	130	150 °C
uPVC	5	6×10^{-5}	75	82 °C
MPVC	5	10×10^{-5}	73	83 °C
GRP	9	40×10^{-6}	89 °C	sustained
Borosilicate glass	0.32	$\times 10^{-5}$		—
Copper	1.7	$\times 10^{-5}$		—
Galvanized steel	1.1	$\times 10^{-5}$		—
Iron	1.0	$\times 10^{-5}$		—

The method of handling and storage of plastic components on site is important as they are 'thermoplastic' and during long periods of strong sunshine (greater than 23 °C) they may soften and distort under load, or when incorrectly supported.

Because they are relatively light they can easily be handled; they should not be thrown about, but stacked carefully. Pipes should be stacked on level flat ground free from stones or other sharp protusions likely to cause damage, and the sockets overhung and laid alternate ends. It is also advisable to protect the ends from damage or unsatisfactory joints may result in test failure.

Some plastics have reduced impact strength in very cold conditions which should be recognized by the installer, and they must not be used to earth electrical equipment and should therefore not be painted as it may disguise the material at some later date.

If they are installed in close proximity to 'hot' services, care must be taken to ensure that there is adequate insulation or space between the systems to prevent softening of the plastic material or drying out of deposited solids in the effluent causing it to adhere to the invert of the pipework. A 25 mm gap is recommended.

Because of their light weight, plastic systems may be prefabricated into large

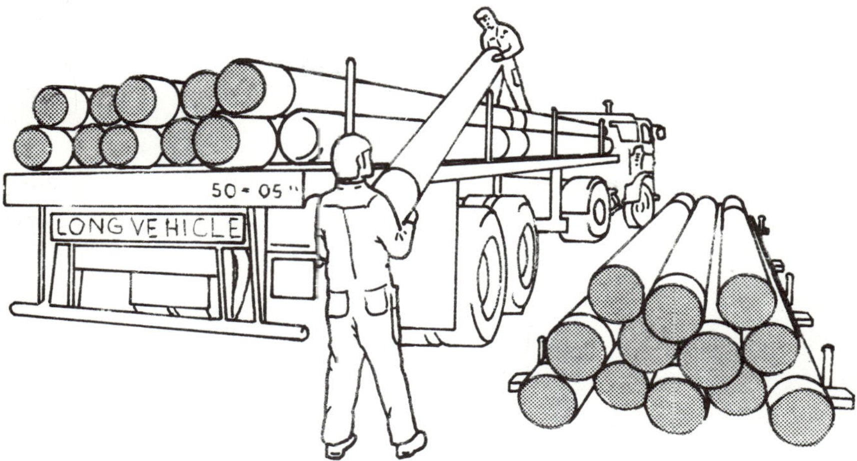

Fig. 4.4 Unplasticized PVC pipes stacked on site

assemblies on the ground before being hoisted up into position in the ceiling zone. Such assemblies can easily be lifted with welded joints, but not so easily with '0' ring joints as they may flop about. Welded systems, however accurately made, may not exactly fit as required, and may therefore be forced or twisted out of their natural shape to compensate for slight inaccuracies. Severe stresses may then be created in the assembly causing eventual failure.

Unplasticized PVC and MPVC is used for most drainage systems, gutters, downpipes and land drains, both above or below ground. Such drainage systems have been well tried and tested over the past 20 years, and those that have been investigated by the Agrément Board have been given a durable life expectancy on excess of 50 years when used in the context of their certificate.

Unplasticized PVC slotted 'french drains' are manufactured for irrigation purposes and land drainage schemes. It is particularly suitable for use in chemically aggressive soils. Pipes are made in sizes from 100 mm to 250 mm nominal bore and in lengths of 6 m and 9 m, one end being socketed.

The slots at right angles into the pipe as it is extruded give a fast rate of infiltration and good flow characteristics. When tested against porous concrete pipes of the same size they showed a marked improvement in their capacity.

When used underground the flexible nature of plastic systems enables them to follow any ground movements that might occur after installation. With more rigid systems fracture of pipework can occur with the consequent risk of blockages developing or the ingress of ground water or tree roots.

This flexibility can also be a disadvantage as, unlike pipes of a more rigid nature where the external loads are supported by the strength of the pipe wall, plastic pipes are capable of considerable circumferential deformation and rely

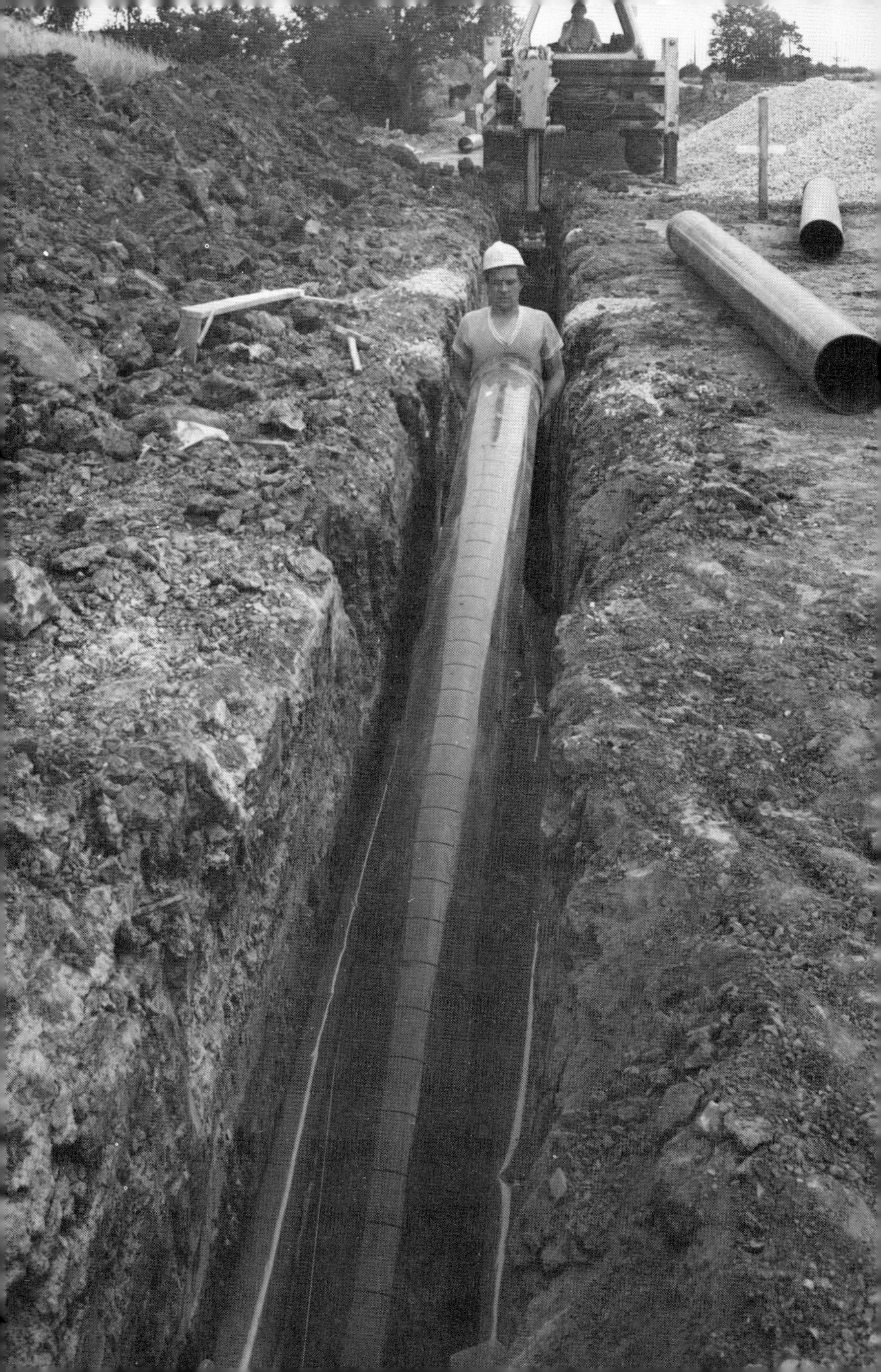

upon keeping their shape by the passive resistance of the surrounding fill.

All plastic systems have special adaptors available to allow them to be connected into systems in other materials.

Glass-reinforced plastic (GRP) pipes and fittings are usually made in large diameters – between 300 and 2000 mm – and are very strong; weight for weight, approximately seven times stronger than steel pipes. But they are also much lighter, therefore they require lighter lifting equipment on site and are also easier to transport than many alternative materials. They can successfully be used in aggressive soils where metal or concrete pipes would be at risk, or for the transportation of many chemical effluents.

Jointing can be undertaken under skilled supervision by semi-skilled operatives and lengths can be cut using hand tools. Because of the very long lengths available there is a reduction in the number of joints and a consequent increase in the speed of laying.

GRP is also used for the manufacture of replacement gutter and downpipe systems for historic buildings where the designer wishes to match the existing cast iron or lead system no longer available.

The jointing of GRP systems can be undertaken by a number of methods, but for non-pressure applications a conventional rolling rubber ring joint is usually specified, but a ridged joint can be formed using a epoxy mortar.

Borosilicate glass

This material is relatively new for drainage purposes, but has been used successfully for chemical processed plant installations for many years. It has the capability of conveying most of the chemical effluents likely to be discharged into a drainage system (except for fluoride solutions), from laboratories and similar establishments, although no information is available on the performance of glass with effluents over 65 °C.

Glass systems in material terms are considerably more expensive than most plastics or clayware systems, but obviously only a small percentage of the total 'as installed' cost. If the client is reluctant to pay this extra cost it would be advisable for the designer to disclaim, in writing, responsibility for any eventual failure through the action of chemicals.

Tests have been carried out to assess the transport performance of 100 mm nominal bore transparent glass pipe using effluent-containing combinations of maternity pads and paper towels flushed into the system via a 'P' trap WC. The performance was found to be between that of unplasticized PVC and spun iron, being closer to unplasticized PVC. For drainage performance calculations the roughness factor can be assumed to be the same as unplasticized PVC.

Glass has been used successfully for both underground and above-ground installations. In the underground system the pipes and fittings are encased in a

Fig. 4.5 (facing page) Laying unplasticized PVC slotted land drain

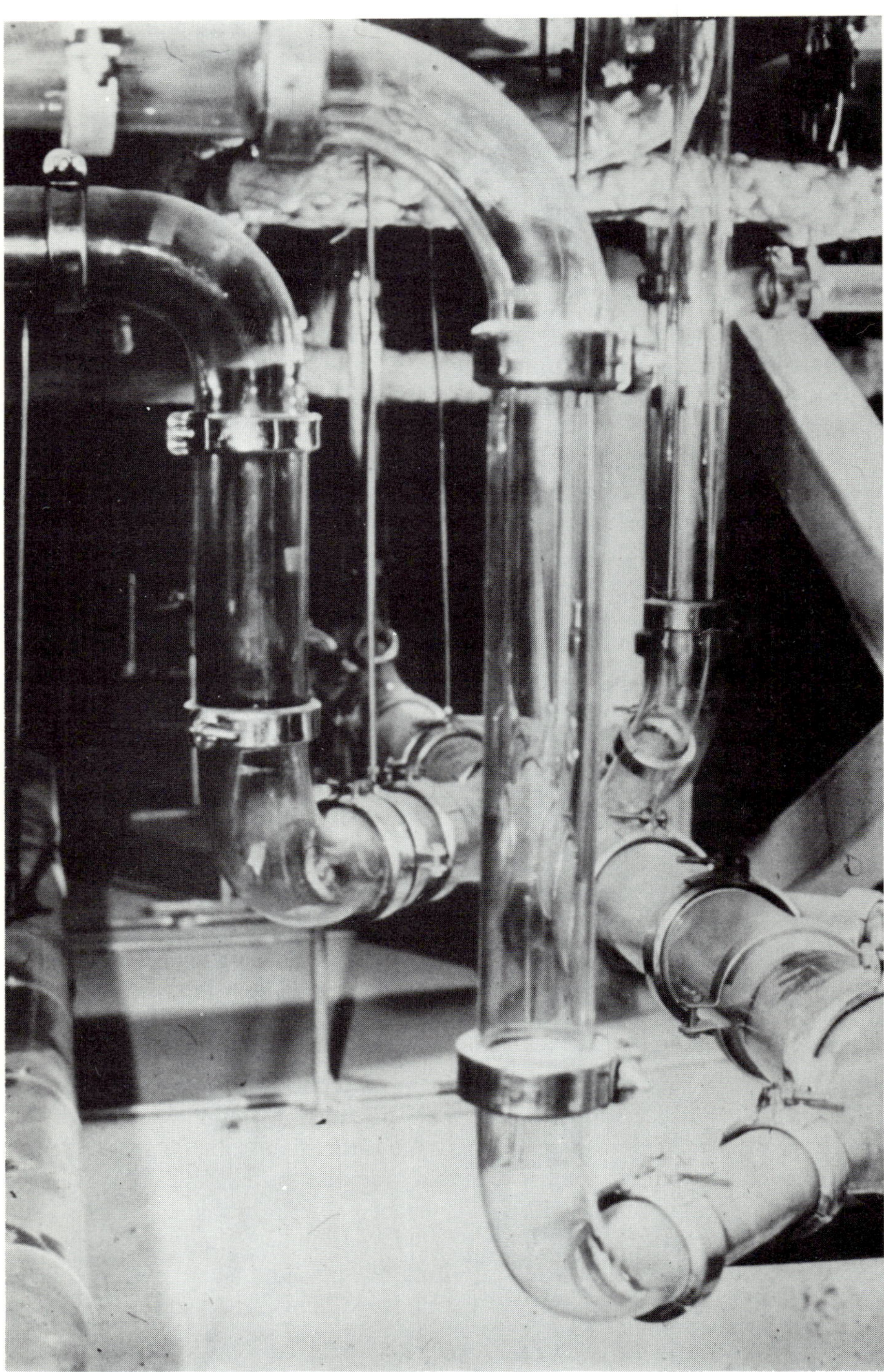

Fig. 4.6 Example of glass drainage

12 mm thick polystyrene jacket as a precaution against impact damage by providing a resilient outer surface. Its impact strength is poor as glass is a brittle material, but it has sufficient strength to withstand normal delivery, handling and stacking loads.

Its thermal movement is very small so that it can be discounted and its performance over a temperature range between 0 °C and 120 °C is excellent; it can also be used in situations down to –20 °C.

It must not however be subjected to thermal shock or it may shatter, and it must be maintained with care as although it is mechanically strong it will shatter under impact. In particular the use of metal-tipped maintenance equipment must be handled with caution.

As the material is rigid and brittle, no movement can be tolerated away from the couplings where up to 4° can be accommodated in all planes.

The jointing of components is by a compression coupling consisting of an outer stainless steel shell tightened by a single stainless steel bolt on to a nitrile rubber liner with a chemically inert PFTE sheath in contact with the effluent.

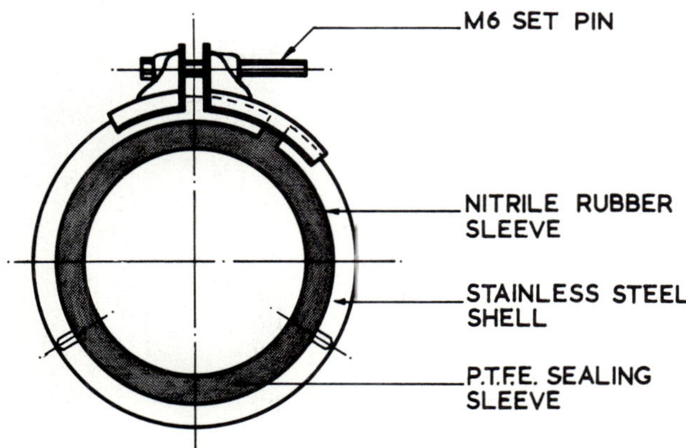

Fig. 4.7 Stainless steel coupling for glass drainage

The external ends of the glass components are beaded, on to which the coupling clamps to form a watertight joint.

Standard pipe lengths are available and it is advisable for designers to work to these dimensions so that cut lengths are kept to a minimum as it is a semi-specialist operation to cut and bead lengths of tube. Although the technique can easily be learnt the equipment is not generally available, consequently quick alterations or repairs to systems cannot readily be undertaken.

Underground drains passing through manholes are provided with sealed access caps, allowing entry for maintenance purposes. Open channels are not available or recommended. By using a sealed system any gases are contained within the pipework, their release being controlled through the vent pipework, thereby obviating any risk of them escaping into areas where people are present.

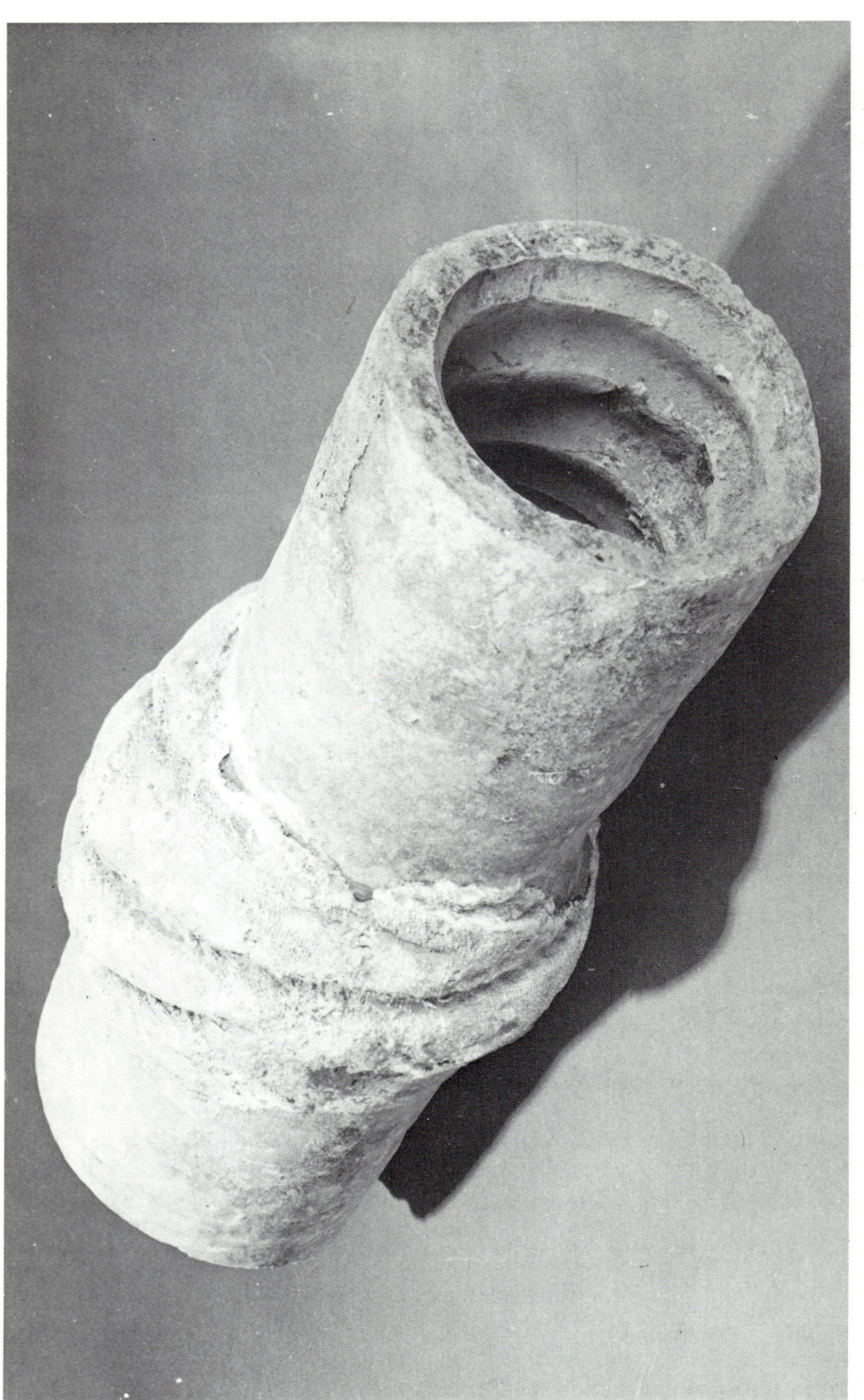

Fig. 4.8 1200-year-old clay pipe excavated in Mecca, Saudi Arabia

Clayware

Traditionally, pipes made from clay have been used underground for drainage purposes for at least 3000 years and their suitability, inherent strength and durability are without question. They cannot be used for above-ground situations or for pipes of less than 75 mm in diameter as they are not manufactured.

Clayware – sometimes called stoneware – pipes and fittings were previously salt-glazed, but this technique is no longer used, being superseded by vitrified clay components which are smoother and denser and can be made to closer tolerances and for pipes of longer length.

Joints between components were traditionally made between an open socket and a spigot by packing in a tarred gasket and then pointing up with a strong

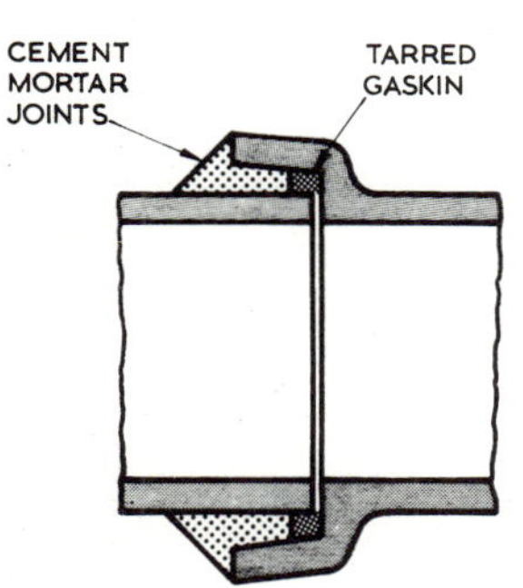

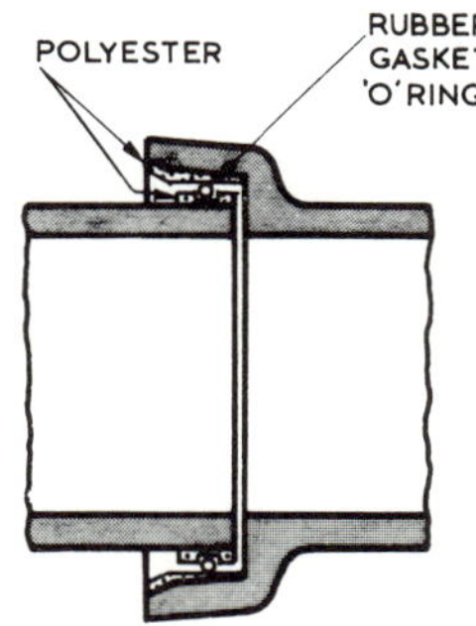

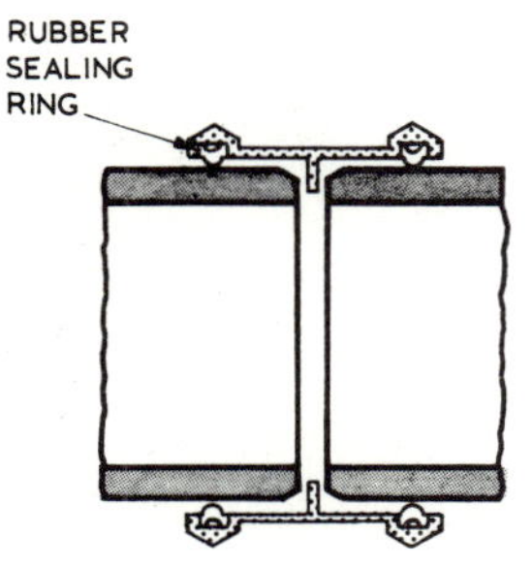

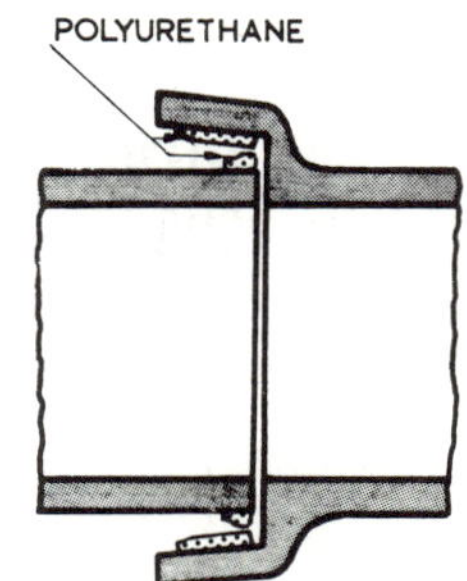

Fig. 4.9 Jointing methods for clayware components

cement mortar which made the whole system a horizontal rigid beam incapable of any movement. Consequently as most soils move (some such as clay by a considerable amount) due to seasonal moisture variations these rigid systems usually break either just behind the collar or at some intermediate point, thereby allowing the ingress of ground water and tree roots. Blockages also occur at these breaks. This method of jointing is inherently inaccurate and lipping of the joints will occur, causing blockages.

Pipes and fittings are still available for use with this type of jointing system, but they are not recommended.

A variety of more acceptable jointing methods are now available for clayware components, all attempting to provide a more accurate method of coupling and flexibility for the system.

Extra long lengths of clayware are now available and they should be used with caution as a beam effect may be created.

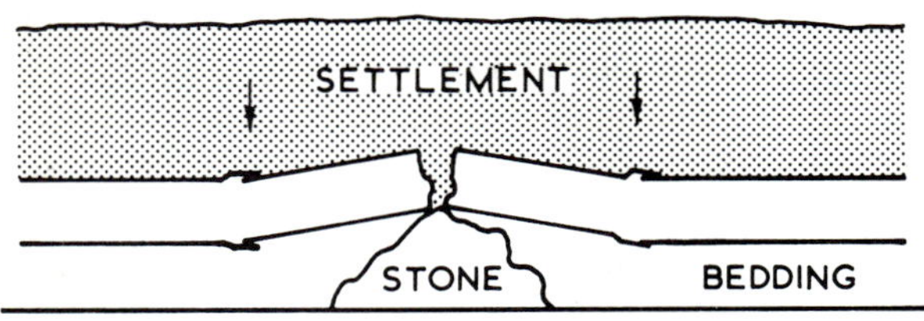

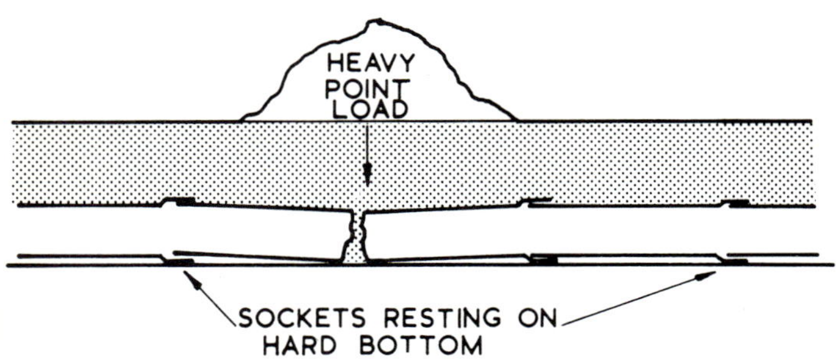

Fig. 4.10 Example of possible breakages

Clayware systems can be used in aggressive soil conditions and for the conveyance of dilute chemical solutions. They are inherently strong and, unlike plastics, do not rely upon the surrounding material to prevent cross sectional deformation under a top load. Because of this strength, they are unyielding and can be easily broken if laid on a protruding hard object or supported on the sockets without adequate packing under the barrel of the pipes.

Clayware systems are available for land drainage with or without plastic couplings.

Iron

Iron pipes and fittings for both above and below ground drainage purposes have traditionally been used for a long time; they have also been used for rainwater gutters and downpipes.

It is a strong and reasonably flexible material which relies upon the total integrity of a bitumen coating to prevent corrosion. It is attacked by the bacteria in certain soil types, aggressive ground water, and chemical effluents.

Iron components are either 'cast' in sand moulds or centrifugally cast (sometimes called spun iron) in metal moulds, a method which produces a better quality product.

The traditional method of jointing sand cast components is by the insertion between the spigot and socket of a tarred hemp gasket and then packing with either cold calked lead wool or hot run molten lead. Asbestos calking compounds are also available for above ground work. If not properly applied the hot lead may penetrate the bore of the pipe with 'fingers', causing blockages to develop.

Lead and cast iron have different coefficients of thermal movement and particularly in ducts or ceiling spaces the joint will in time break down and weep effluent.

It has been known for the bitumen coating to fill 'blow holes' in poor castings, and although the system will stand a test the bitumen may melt out with very hot discharges.

Sand casting is a crude method of manufacture and drainage components so made do not comply with the performance standards laid down here, or in Codes of Practice.

These criteria are that the components must be

(a) Of smooth bore.
(b) Well radiused.
(c) Joints that accurately align the components.

Research and experience has shown that more blockages occur in cast iron drainage systems due to the material than in any other system, particularly if multi-branch junctions have been used.

It is not advisable to use sand cast iron for foul drainage systems.

Centrifugally cast or spun iron pipes are of much better quality than those manufactured by the sand casting method and can be used with some confidence.

The jointing of components is carried out in a similar manner to the glass system. A cast iron split coupling is pulled together on to a synthetic rubber gasket by two stainless steel bolts. The spigot ends of fittings are beaded, but as the pipes have doubled spigotted plain ends, square cut lengths can therefore be

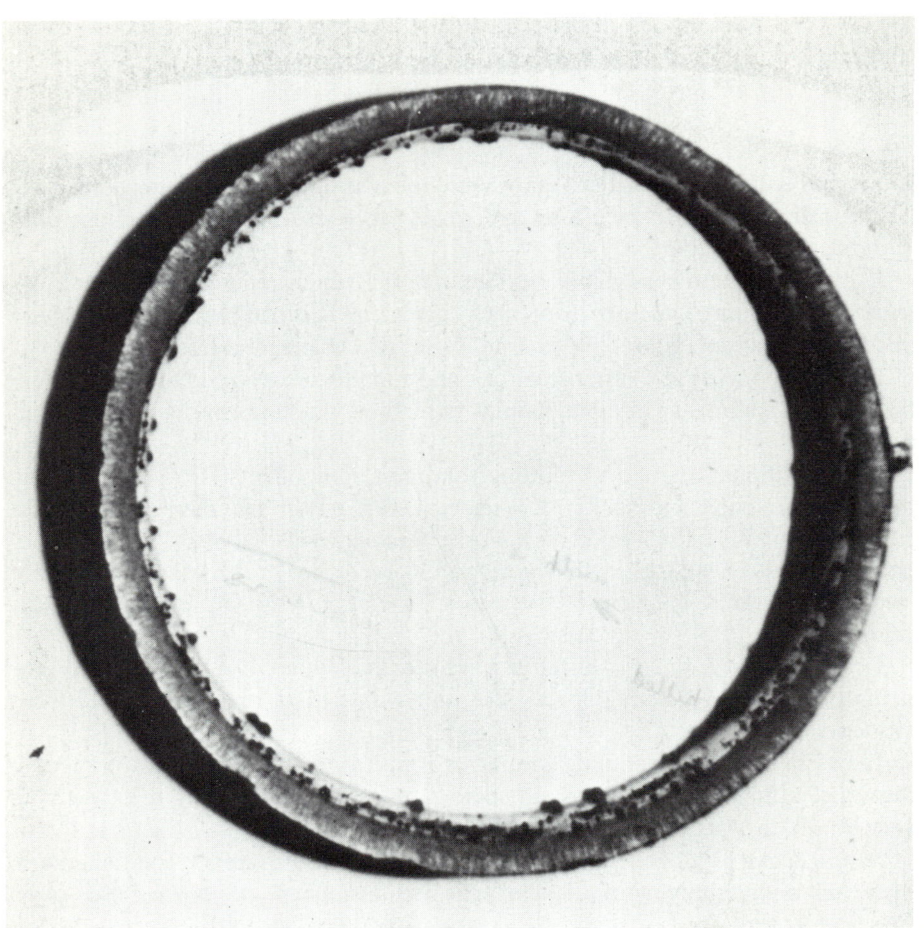

Fig. 4.11 Section through rough bore cast iron pipe

utilized. Because the pipe lacks the bead it is not preset in the coupling and the installer must ensure it is fully pushed home.

It is a strong flexible system and is of great use where mechanical damage may be a problem or where very high temperature discharges are likely.

Copper

The use of copper as a drainage material is usually confined to wastes up to 42 mm in diameter, but because of its relatively high cost is often only specified for quality installations or where high-temperature discharges such as from kitchen equipment are likely to be experienced.

Copper systems can only be used in above-ground situations and as the pipework, fittings and jointing systems (either capillary solder or mechanical compression) meet the performance requirements blockages are unlikely. Knuckle

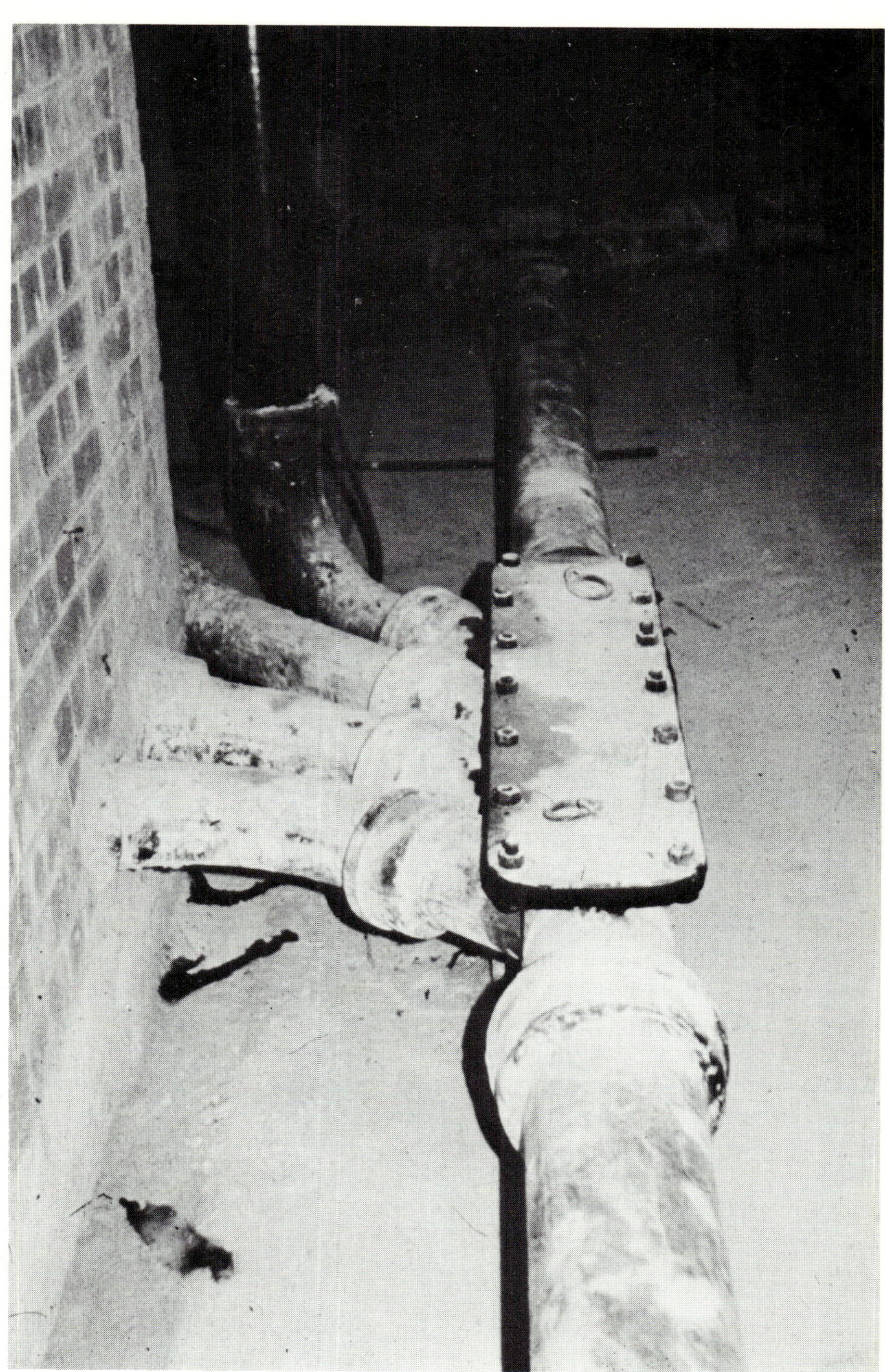

Fig. 4.12 Cast iron multi-branch junction

bends and right angle junctions should not be used.

Copper is particularly useful for repetitive prefabrication of preplumbed units in service ducts where site installation can be quickly undertaken as the major part of the installation is carried out off the site.

Fittings are often in brass or gun metal and are available for jointing copper wastes into iron components.

Galvanized mild steel

Galvanized mild steel is used only for above-ground drainage systems and often for prefabricated assemblies. Tests undertaken by the Building Research Station indicate that no significant loss of zinc will occur due to use.

Prefabricated assemblies are made up from steel tube plate or angles butt welded together and zinc galvanized after fabrication by a hot dip process that coats both the inside and outside of the system.

To joint assemblies together a calking socket is made with a collar at least 25 mm larger than the pipe it is to receive and the manufacturers recommend the use of a cold calking compound. Butt welding can leave protrusions into the bore of the pipework and an examination should be carried out before installation.

Concrete

Concrete underground drainage systems are manufactured in sizes between 150 mm and 1200 mm diameter and are recommended for use in surface and storm water drainage schemes; they are also available for land drains.

They should not be used for the conveyance of even lightly charged chemical effluents, or where the soil the system is to be installed in contains sulphates in the ground water.

Sulphates occur mainly in the clay stratas; London Clay, Lower Lias, Oxford Clay, Kimmeridge Clay and Keuper Marl. They can also occur in made-up grounds formed from brick rubble, ash and some industrial wastes. The rate of sulphate attack will depend on the quality of the concrete (its permeability) and the amount and nature of the sulphates present in the ground. It must be stated that although concrete pipes may appear vulnerable to sulphate attack they are usually manufactured from a high quality concrete; the attack therefore may be minimal. If sulphates are present the designer should consider using another material such as GRP for the larger sizes or unplasterized PVC or clayware for sizes up to 300 mm.

Lead and asbestos coment, and pitch fibre

These materials are still available for drainage purposes but have mainly been superseded by alternatives which have better overall performance characteristics.

Chapter 5

Components

Introduction

The components listed in the index are those commonly found as part of a drainage system. It must be the designer's prerogative to select which manufacturer's product to use but some guidance is given to assist in the choice of components and their function.

Components must fulfill their function economically and in a satisfactory manner; they must not cause blockages to develop, or release effluent. If a blockage does occur they must not impede the maintenance operator's task of cleansing and they must not create a hazard to health and safety.

Manholes and inspection chambers

There are various interpretations of these two terms, but the Building Regulations only acknowledge the existence of the latter, although the British Standard Code of Practice refers to both types of chamber.

The regulations define an inspection chamber as 'any chamber constructed on a drain so as to provide access for inspection and cleansing'. Various other documents add to this definition the words 'and the removal of debris when operating from surface level,' and, related to manholes, 'permitting man entry'.

Whichever definition you prefer, the objective of either chamber is to provide adequate access into the drainage system for testing and maintenance.

The siting of such chambers is set out in various statutory documents as follows:

(a) At each point in a drainage system where there is a change in gradient or direction which would prevent any part of the system being readily cleansed without such a chamber.

    Unfortunately this is taken to mean that any deviation from a straight line must have a chamber, although it is easily possible to clean a drain with modern equipment when it is laid to a gradual curve.

(b) Within 12.5 m from a junction between drains if there is no chamber at the junction.

As all junctions are inherently changes in direction (a), there must always be a chamber at a junction, and as such junctions may precipitate blockages this reasoning is very sound when open channels are used; but where a junction is formed by a well-made 45° pipe fitting, blockages are unlikely.

(c) At the top end of a drainage system if there is no rodding point.

(d) 90 m apart; or that no part of a drainage system shall be at a distance of more than 45 m from a chamber

It is difficult to understand how this arbitrary distance was arrived at although it is professed by very old maintenance operatives that 45 m is about the maximum distance a set of cane rods can be pushed up – or down – a surcharged 110 mm drain. Specialist drain-cleaning companies, however, maintain that mechanically powered rods can easily and effectively travel at least 200 m in either direction.

In May 1954 a report based upon an extensive survey was issued by the Joint Committee on Field Research into Drainage Problems. It attempted to identify the reasons why blockages develop in underground drainage systems. There were fourteen basic causes outlined as well as the general cause of misuse; two of the reasons were:

(a) Faulty design of invert channels in manholes; branches have sometimes been brought in at too acute an angle against the flow of the main channel.

(b) Defective construction of manholes including unsuitable bricks and covers and poor rendering.

It also states that it is evident from the information obtained (from the survey) that the part of the drainage system at which most blockages occur is the interceptor.

Figure 5.1 shows an inspection chamber and interceptor trap, the latter being fitted with a flanged cleaning arm and cover, a second cover giving access to the trap. A side socket is provided for the connection to a fresh air inlet.

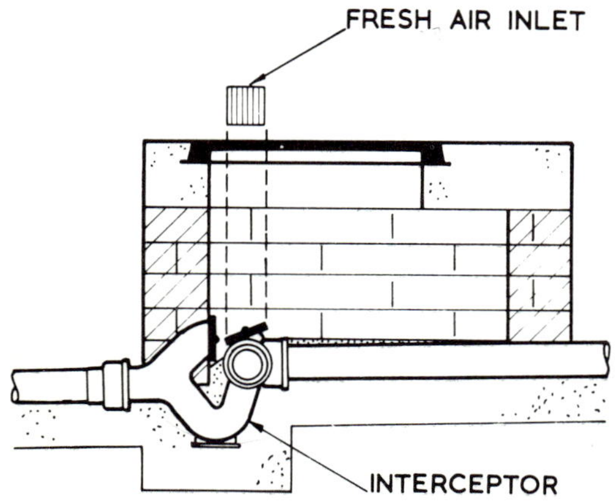

Fig. 5.1 Standard arrangement for an interceptor trap

Further surveys have shown that open channel chambers and those containing cast iron multibranch junctions are more likely to develop blockages than chambers containing a sealed system of junction fittings in a smooth bore material such as PVC.

Acute branch channel bends turn a drain into the direction of the main flow, but in so doing prevent adequate access up the incoming drain and are a known cause of blockages; 140° and 165° channel bends should not be used in foul systems.

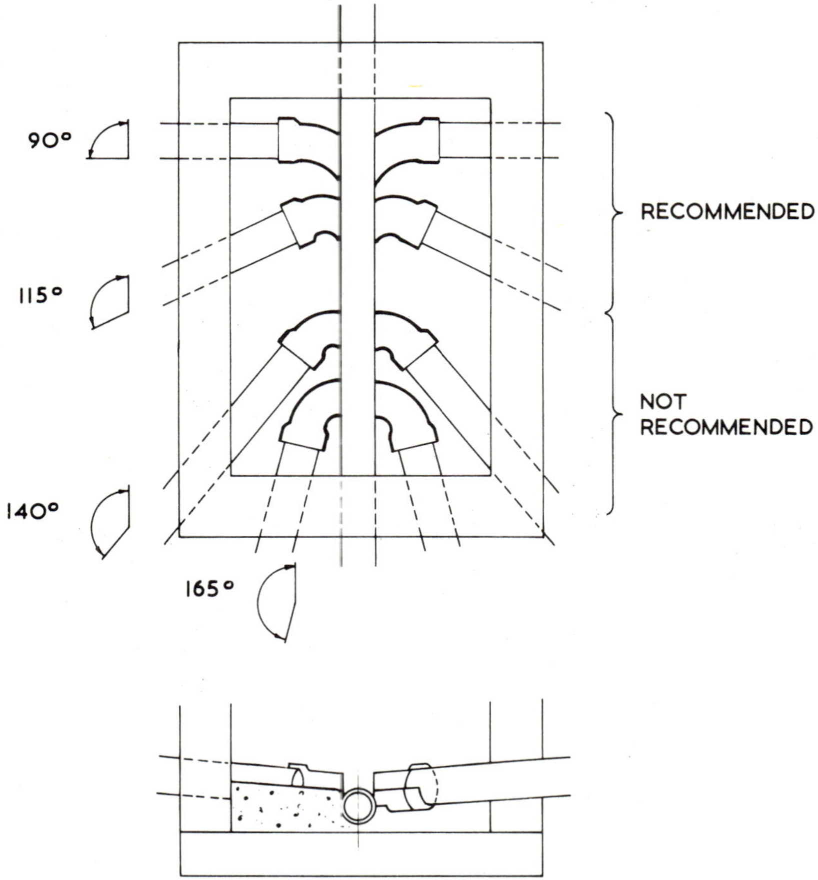

Fig. 5.2 Chamber junctions liable to cause blockage

All chambers must be capable of:

(a) Sustaining the load that may be imposed upon them; this is particularly important when the chamber is shallow and in an area where heavy vehicles may pass over them.

(b) Being watertight against both external and internal water pressure.

(c) Permitting ready and easy access for testing, inspection and maintenance.
(d) Having a removable non-ventilating cover of adequate strength and durability, but when situated internally within a building the whole cover construction including the frame must be water tight when subjected to an internal pressure which would develop if a blockage occurred down stream of the chamber.
(e) Covers on internal chambers must also be air tight and secured to the frame by removable bolts made of non-corrosive material.
(f) When the drain inverts within a chamber are too deep to be reached easily from the ground the walls must be fitted with step irons or ladders to provide safe access to the level of the pipework.
(g) If open channels are to be used the base of the chamber must be provided with benching having a smooth impervious finish and so formed to provide a safe foothold and to guide the flow of effluent from all the branches towards the outfall from the chamber.
(h) All branches entering a chamber should be formed so that the effluent is directed obliquely into the direction of flow. An angle of 45° is recommended.
(i) Channel bends should have their inverts set above that of the through drain channel to prevent backing up, and if possible should not be sited diagonally opposite each other.
(j) Sealed pipework systems must have means of draining the chamber into the system.

One recommended method is by the provision of an easily removable standing plug.

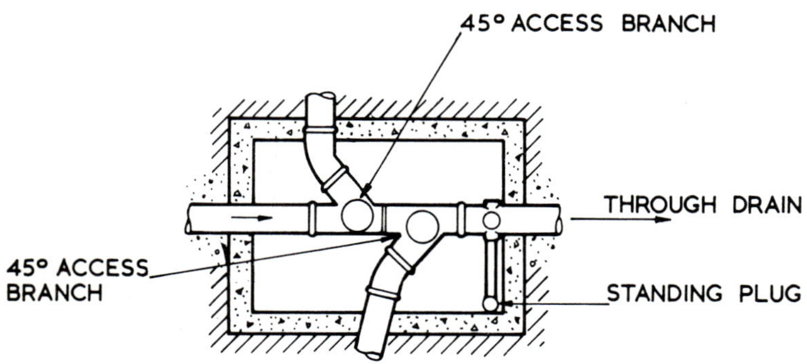

Fig. 5.3 Recommended pipework arrangement

The designer of drainage systems should endeavour to set out the schemes in such a manner as to reduce the number of chambers to a minimum, but on no account should he attempt to bring together branch drains into one chamber in such a manner that will precipitate blockages or effectively prevent the maintenance of any branch.

Inspection chambers and manholes are relatively expensive components within the total system, and therefore their specification should be limited to the minimum necessary to provide adequate access into the system. Rodding points should be used wherever possible, but there must always be a chamber positioned where items may be taken out of the system.

Great care must be taken in positioning internal chambers and the designer must always be aware that during maintenance they may release pathogens into the internal areas. In particular internal chambers in hospitals, kitchens or food preparation areas should be avoided.

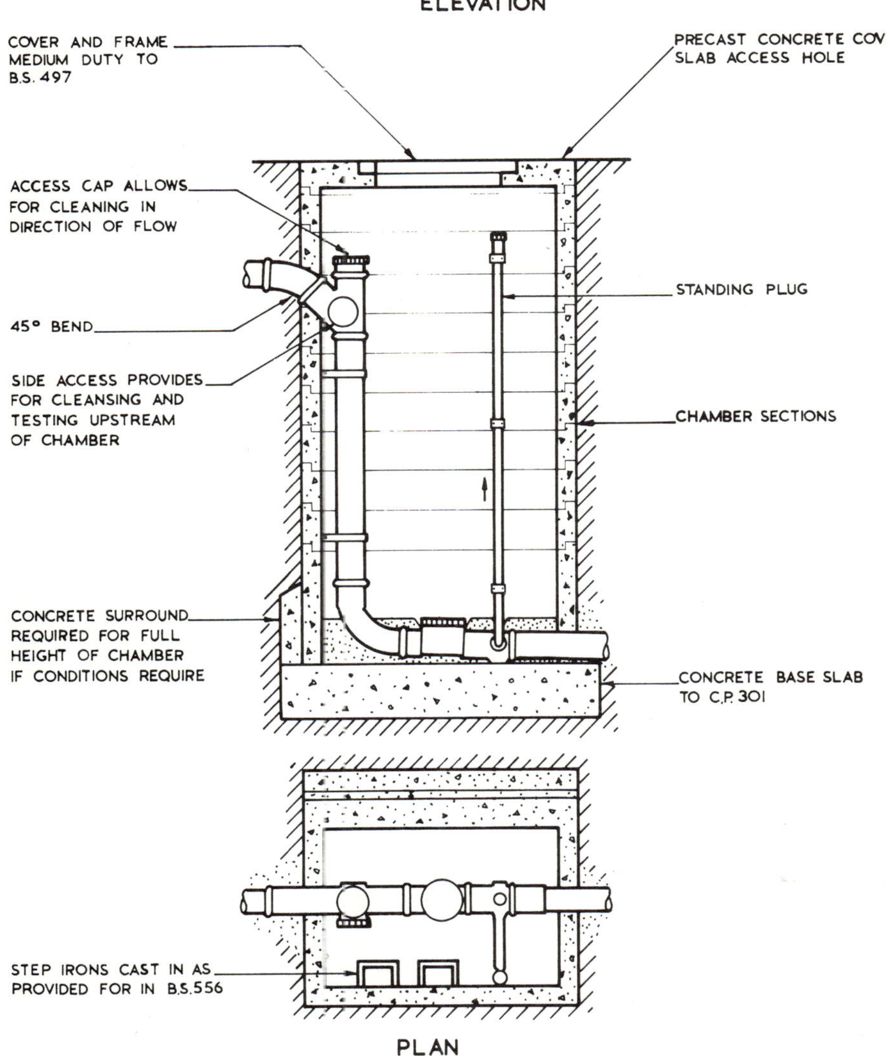

Fig. 5.4 Typical back drop chamber

Open channel chambers are liable to gradual deterioration due to the action of the gases and effluents and therefore require planned maintenance – the more chambers the greater the cost of the maintenance.

Manufacturer's catalogues show chamber configurations which are sometimes taken by the unknowing as tacit approval for the use of acute channel junctions or multibranch junctions, but experience has shown that some of these examples should not be used in practice.

The gradient of a drainage system should be as flat as allowable under the hydraulic design rules, and where possible should follow the ground contours.

If deep manholes are necessary to meet the invert of an existing drain or sewer, back drops should be used rather than increase the gradient of the drain – excavation costs money.

It is preferred that such back drops should be internal to the chamber as the quality of workmanship can be observed and backfilling or settlement will not disturb the pipework. The change from horizontal drain to vertical drop should be by the use of a 45° bend and junction, and the bend at the base of the drop should be of large radius.

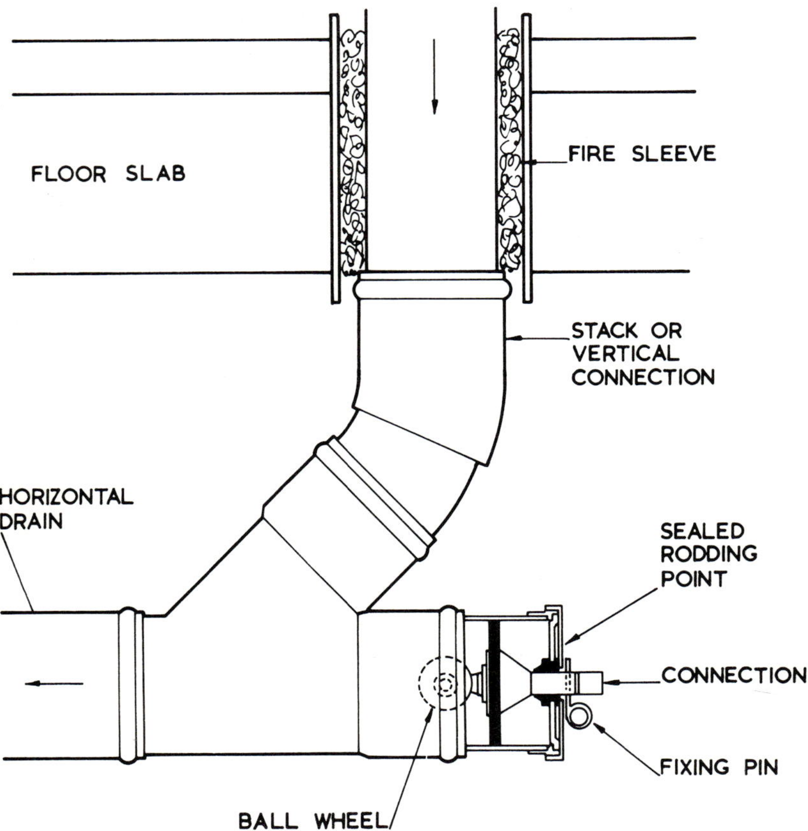

Fig. 5.5 Sealed rodding point

Rodding points

Rodding points can usefully be employed internally within a building drainage system in place of the more traditional access fittings, or externally at the head of a drain or branch. They are particularly appropriate for use in undercrofts or basements as sealed points where opening a blocked drain would otherwise result in flooding.

The cleaning device is permanently in position in the rodding point so that to bring it into operation only requires the connection of the rod a continuous coil of plastic, the removal of the fixing pin. The whole can then be progressed along the pipe. After the drain has been cleansed the rod head is brought back and the pin replaced so that the rod can be disconnected.

The risk of flooding is thus obviated and there is also little risk of contamination from the cleaning operation.

All rodding points should be connected into the drainage system using 45° fittings in the direction of the main flow. They should be at least 110 mm in diameter and preferably of the same size as the drain into which they are connected.

When a stack junction into a horizontal drain is over 6 m from the next chamber it is advisable to position a rodding point near to the base of the stack.

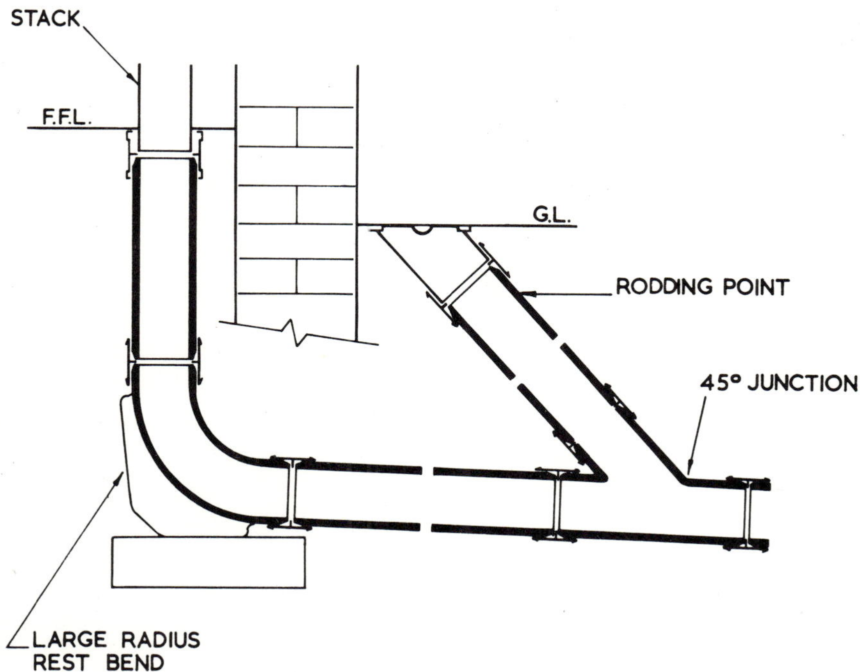

Fig. 5.6 Rodding point near base of stack

Gullies

Gullies on foul drainage systems are small septic tanks giving ideal conditions for the growth of bacteria and should not be used internally in hospitals where the risk of contamination cannot be tolerated.

It is unnecessary to double trap sanitary appliances; any appliance that has its own associated trap can discharge directly into the drainage system. Waste appliances do not have to be connected into a sealed side or back inlet gully, but should discharge through a standing waste with rodding facility at either the trap or top of the waste.

Macerators should not discharge over gullies even from a ground floor kitchen when the sink is on an external wall.

Road gullies should have access points to allow the clearing of silt deposits from the surface water drains.

Yard gullies and those gullies provided for wash down facilities for vehicle parks, etc., should be provided with grit buckets to prevent and collect surface detritus passing into the drainage system. Such gullies will require regular maintenance, the time interval dependent upon the washing procedure and amount of dirt collected.

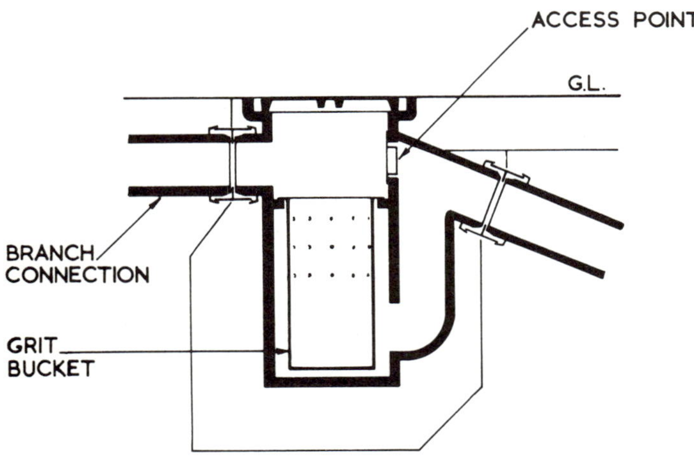

Fig. 5.7 Yard gully with branch connection and access point

Mud sump

Any surface water or land drain that is likely to carry sedimentary deposits of silt, sand or grit must be connected into a mud sump prior to discharging into a combined or main surface water drain.

Such drains should have a rodding point at the head of the drain to enable the system to be cleaned out at planned intervals so that they can continue to be effective. Land drains in particular, by their nature, tend to become blocked in time by the deposit of silt and must therefore be subjected to periodic maintenance.

Grease interceptors/traps

In general grease interceptors should not be installed into a drainage system even where mass catering establishments such as factory or hospital kitchens are concerned.

Animal grease is little used in kitchens, being replaced by vegetable oils which cannot be isolated by such interceptors or traps.

Grease may enter the drainage system via food waste macerators which, by using only cold water, enable it to pass through the pipework system. It may also enter the system from automatic dish-washing equipment, but is emulsified by the very hot water and detergents used.

If grease interceptors are to be specified the following rules apply:

(a) They should be placed in the drainage system in such a manner that they do not receive foul sewage waste; only grease should be collected.

(b) They should be sited in a position where the effluent temperature will allow cooling to deposit the grease within the chamber.

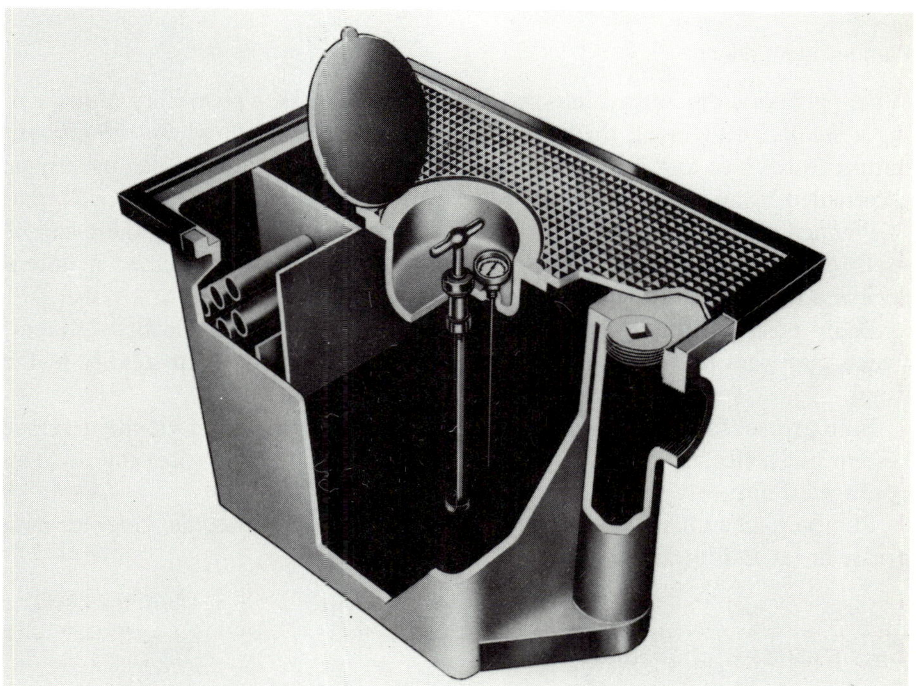

Fig. 5.8 Biological degrading grease interceptor

(c) The chamber must have adequate capacity to effectively allow the entering grease to cool and remain therein.
(d) Detergents or the effluent from dishwashers should not be discharged into such chambers.
(e) Regular and frequent planned maintenance will be required to remove the solidified grease. This is an obnoxious task and is therefore often neglected.

There are available non-mechanical grease interceptors that break down the grease by biochemical action. They must be regularly dosed with proprietary chemicals in solution which then attacks the grease and allows it to be flushed through the system.

The temperature of the contents of these interceptors must not exceed 43 °C and chlorine or strong caustics must not enter the system; but diluted they can be considered acceptable.

These interceptors are able to process effectively the normal discharge of waste water with grease in suspension, but are not capable of digesting oil or grease in concentration and they will not deal with any type of mineral oil.

The discharge of food waste with grease via macerators is not recommended to pass into this type of equipment as there will inevitably be a build-up of sediment and unacceptable maintenance implications.

Dosing procedures must be carried out in strict accordance with the component manufacturer's instructions.

Planned maintenance

Where grease is discharged into the drains there may be a possibility of it forming a solid coating along the bore of the drain from a point where the effluent temperature cools to a degree where solidification can occur; this can usually be ascertained by an inspection of the manholes along the line of the drain.

Planned maintenance by either scraping through or chemical cleaning can be used to cleanse the system. Grease interceptors also require planned maintenance and there is some commercial value of the grease recovered.

Badly positioned interceptors may not sufficiently cool the loaded effluent, which may pass through the chamber, and the grease may then solidify in the drain.

Bulk grease, fat or old cooking oils should not be disposed of via the drainage system but collected in containers and removed for either reprocessing or to an approved dump.

Pumping chambers and associated equipment will become clogged with grease or fat and interceptors will be required.

Septic tanks and cesspools

A septic tank is a method of sewage disposal for buildings that cannot be

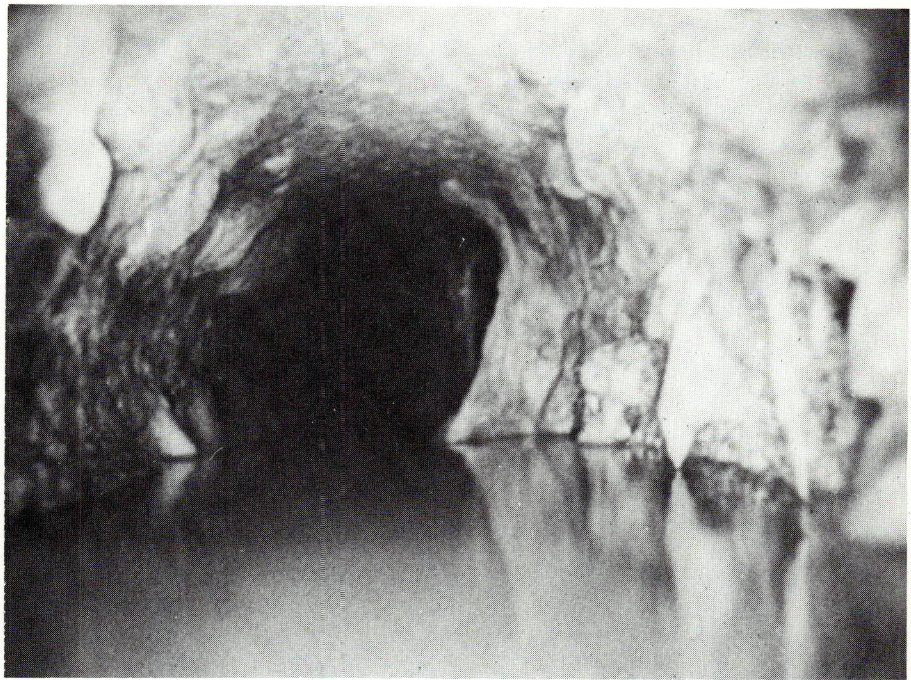

Fig. 5.9 Grease build-up inside drain

coupled into a main sewage drainage system. It is a tank through which sewage is passed to settle the solid contents held in suspension in the conveying water which are retained in the tank to undergo digestion by anaerobic bacterial action. The liquid after settlement is dissipated into the surrounding ground via a land drainage pipework network.

Tanks should be sized upon the basis of the number of persons likely to use the associated sanitary appliances, although this is a variable method as it does not take into account visitors, or long period of absences by the occupiers as may occur by the owners of second homes or holiday dwellings.

Desludging by the removal of the settled solids should be carried out every twelve months, although this period may be extended depending upon the frequency of use of the appliances. Dual flush cisterns of WCs and showers will reduce the flow into the tank; surface water should not enter the system.

They are usually sized on the basis that each occupant of the associated dwelling will use 180 litres of water per day, added to a basic capacity of 2000 litres. If a sink macerator is installed 70 litres per person should be added. It can be an advantage to fit a water meter to monitor the quantities used as this will give a more accurate guide to the periods of time between desludging, a relatively expensive operation in country areas.

The waste water run off from the tank is allowed to percolate through the land drainage system – which must be provided with access for maintenance – into the surrounding ground after the solids have settled out. To assist this action, tanks should be fitted with baffles. Biological digestion usually reduces the solids to about one-third of their original volume.

Most local authorities will supply a design drawing of their approved septic tank, usually based upon British Standard Code of Practice (CP302) Small Sewage Treatment Works. The recommended construction is traditional in concept, but the performances specification requires a watertight structure including the base and walls, capable of supporting the load of the tank and its contents, and resistant to ground movement and internal and external water pressures.

In certain respects the land drainage network is more important than the septic tank for if it fails to dissipate the liquid discharged or acts in reverse the tank will overflow.

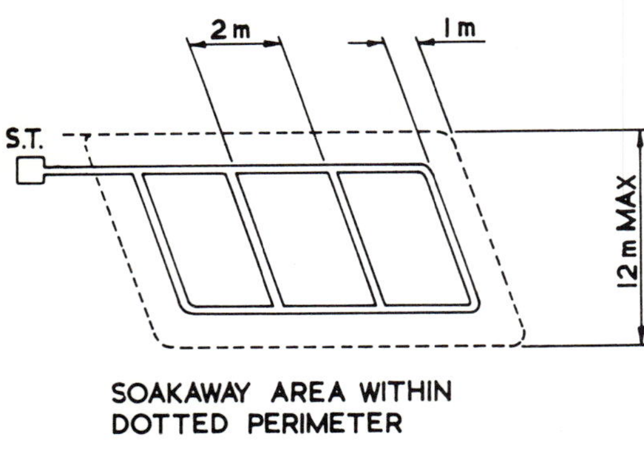

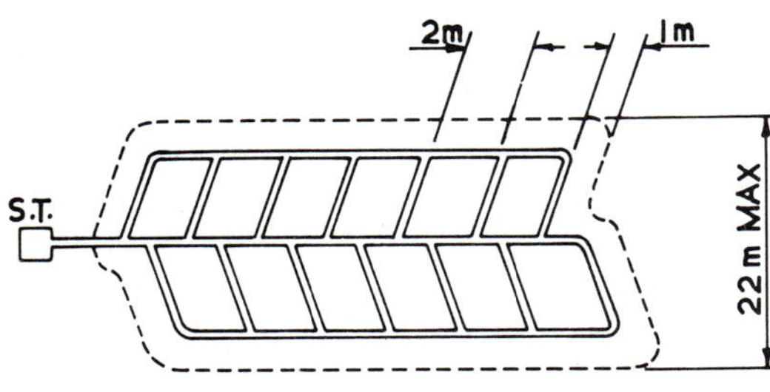

Fig. 5.10 Land drainage systems

The suitability of the ground into which it is proposed to lay the land drainage network must be investigated and the following taken into account.

(a) Clay soils are unsuitable as the liquid would not percolate away, but remain in the network.

(b) The network may fill and even flood back into the tank if the ground water table is high. This should be checked by the trial hole method in both winter and summer.
(c) If it is to be laid in agricultural ground it may be liable to damage by tractors moving or deep ploughing.
(d) Is water collected for drinking purposes downhill of the proposed network? In some country areas wells are still in use.
(e) The liquid would form an ideal feed for tree or shrub roots and the network would soon become clogged if sited in the vicinity of trees. Little trees grow bigger; a rough guide is that the spread of the root system may be horizontally as extensive as the height of the tree.

An ideal site for the network is under a free draining lawn or paddock where it will not be disturbed. It should be laid at a depth of about 250 mm minimum to the crown of the 110 mm pipe and slope at a gentle gradient of about 1 in 200 so that the liquid does not flow quickly to the far end of the system, but is dissipated evenly along the length of the network.

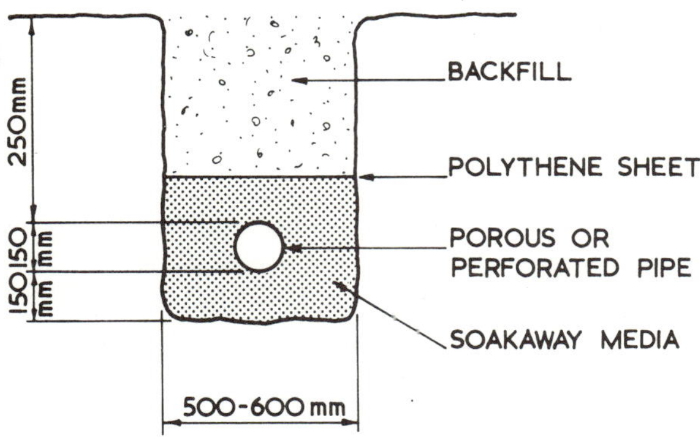

Fig. 5.11 Section through land drain

Tanks should not be sited within 15 m of habitable buildings, although some authorities require a greater distance. They should not be positioned in driveways or positions where they can be physically damaged by heavy vehicles; a minimum distance of 2 m is recommended.

All septic tanks must have adequate access covers for maintenance purposes and a fresh air inlet fitting; dip tubes are useful for plumbing the depth of the deposit.

Glass Reinforced Plastic (GRP) tanks are now available and offer certain advantages over the more traditional forms of construction. They are quickly installed and relatively light in weight. All that is required is a hole of adequate size and depth with a 150 mm layer of granular fill as a base. The tank is then lowered into position and backfilled with similar material. Excavated material should only be used if it is free flowing and free from lumps, large stones or anything which may damage the walls of the tank.

The backfill should be placed in a similar manner as in trench work, i.e. in layers 150 mm thick and lightly compacted to ensure that there are no hollow pockets.

On temporary construction sites after completion of the works these tanks may be emptied and removed fore-use.

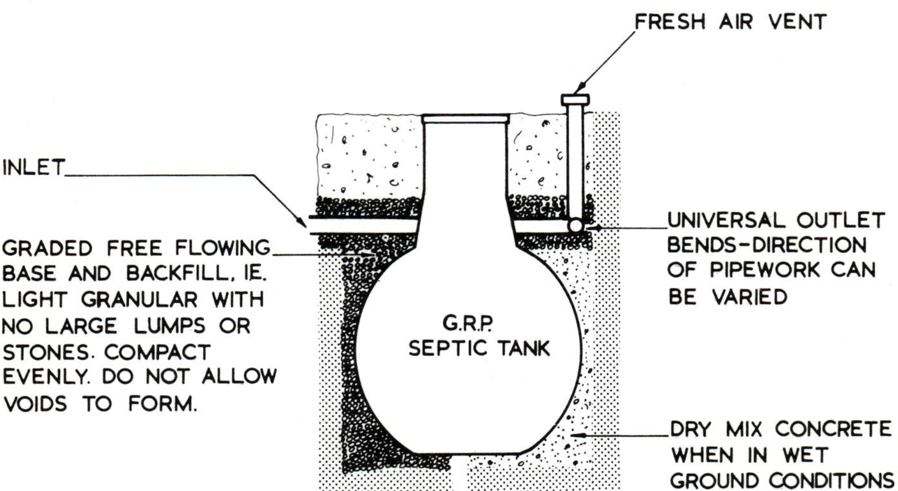

Fig. 5.12 GRP septic tank

As the tanks are light, flotation may be a problem, and they should be partially filled with water during installation if necessary.

Planned maintenance

If the solids are not periodically removed from the tank there is a risk that the sump or land drainage network will become choked, requiring expensive cleaning or complete reinstatement. They require emptying about once a year, but good practice dictates that some sludge must be left in the tank to restart the bacteriological process of digestion.

During maintenance the inside of the tank should be hosed down, including access shafts and dip pipes. The covers should be checked and new grease inserted into the joint between the frame. It is very important that the fresh air inlet is checked and put in good working order. If there is any possibility of these valves being damaged by animals or children they should be raised to a level where they will be out of harm's way.

Cesspools are watertight sealed tanks holding the total foul outflow from the building. They require emptying at regular periods and should only be used when mains drainage is not available or septic tanks cannot be installed – usually because of the ground required for the land drainage network.

Petrol interceptors

Section 27 of the 1936 Public Health Act states that no person shall dispose of any petroleum spirit as prescribed by the Petroleum (Consolidation) Act of 1928 into any drain or sewer communicating with a public sewer.

Many authorities do not require petrol interceptors to be provided in the surface water drainage system from external car parks as they consider that the volatile nature of petroleum will ensure that it will evaporate before it reaches the sewer system; but if oil spillage is likely interceptors are essential.

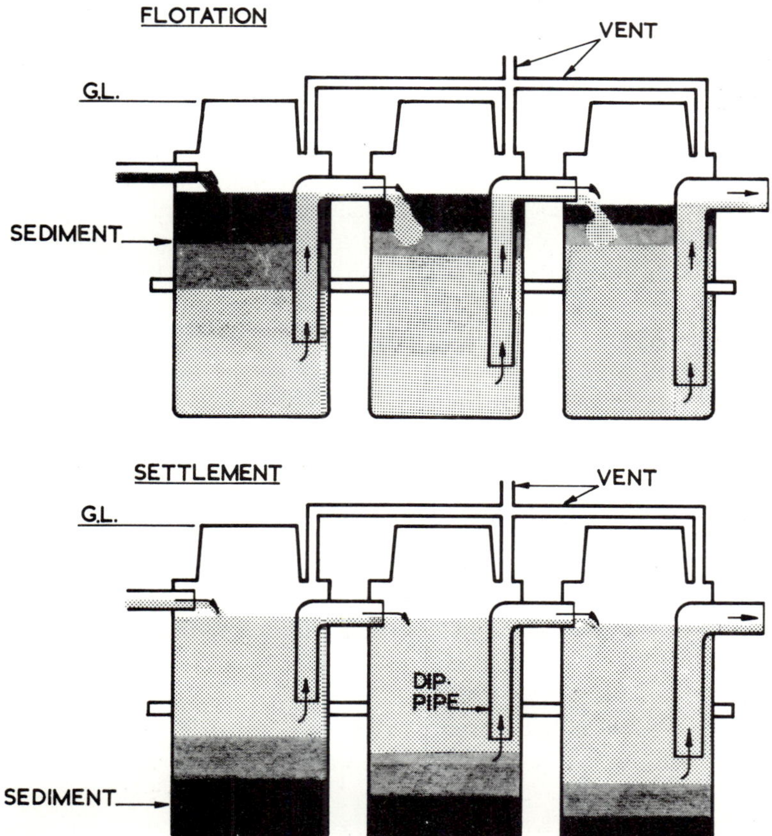

Fig. 5.13 GRP petrol/oil interceptor

Internal car parks should always have petrol interceptors sited away from the building on the surface water system.

The whole of such a drainage system should be well ventilated, including the interceptor. Each section of the interceptor should have a ventilation pipe taken either separately or cross connected and taken up to a minimum height of 2.5 m above ground level and not less than 1.0 m above the height of any adjacent window opening and at a horizontal distance of at least 3.0 m – the top of which should be provided with a secure grille to prevent the ingress of birds, leaves, etc., which may block the outlet.

Traditionally petrol interceptors are constructed in a similar manner as septic tanks or manholes. They are usually three-part chambers, each part interlinked and ventilated. The objective is to break up the inflowing water to release any petroleum spirits or oil held in suspension and hold them until they have evaporated away, or settled out and can be collected.

Pollutants that are lighter than water float to the surface of the liquid held in the tank, but heavy oils mixed with solids may settle to the bottom and have to be removed. The same tank can be used for both methods of pollution control, but the dip pipes must be cut back for the collection of heavy pollutants.

Such an interceptor is essential for garage forecourts, vehicle bays and fuel distribution areas, but to reduce the quantity of solids that may find their way into the chambers grit buckets should be fitted into all gullies.

As with the installation of GRP septic tanks, flotation may be a problem during installation and should be dealt with by partially filling the tank with water. As it is likely that these tanks may be subjected to heavy vehicles moving over or in close proximity to them, they should be surrounded in concrete and protected by a reinforced concrete slab. Heavy duty covers must be specified.

All vent pipes should have a gradual slope back to the chamber to prevent air locks occurring. Vent pipework above ground must not be in plastic, which could easily be broken.

Planned maintenance

All such chambers should be cleaned out annually and the vent pipework inspected.

Maintenance within the chamber must be carried out with extreme caution as the chemical fumes may be toxic. Smoking must not be allowed during this exercise.

Chapter 6

Practical hydraulics

Introduction

Potable water flows through the pipework system within our buildings a full bore either from the mains supply, a storage tank situated in the roof space or from a pump.

The flow of effluent in a drainage system is however usually caused by the force of gravity, as all liquids will attempt to find their own level. Effluent discharged from appliances will therefore flow downhill, the velocity of this flow depending upon a number of factors, but in simple terms the steeper the gradient the greater the velocity and consequently the greater the capacity of the pipework. The velocity and capacity are also controlled to some degree by the roughness of the material and the number of restrictions to free flow such as bends, junctions and manholes, etc.

The discharge from a single appliance entering a drain or stack will soon clear the system, leaving it empty – except for air at atmospheric pressure – and any flow through the system must displace this air. The action of the flow will also draw air into the pipework system, either through the appliance discharging or through the open end of the stack or vent.

These variations in air movement, if not properly controlled, can cause the appliance trap seals to be sucked out by 'siphonage' or blown back by 'back pressure' with the consequence that drain air may enter the building or unacceptable noise may be created.

It is advisable to design stacks and drains to flow only partially full for reasons that will be explained later), and this flow will therefore cause substantial fluctuations in both air pressure and movement through a system.

Pressure limitations

The amount of air movement within a pipework system can be controlled to within acceptable levels by a number of methods.

(a) Ventilation pipework – to allow the free movement of air to each appliance outlet – was traditionally provided, thereby doubling the amount of pipe-

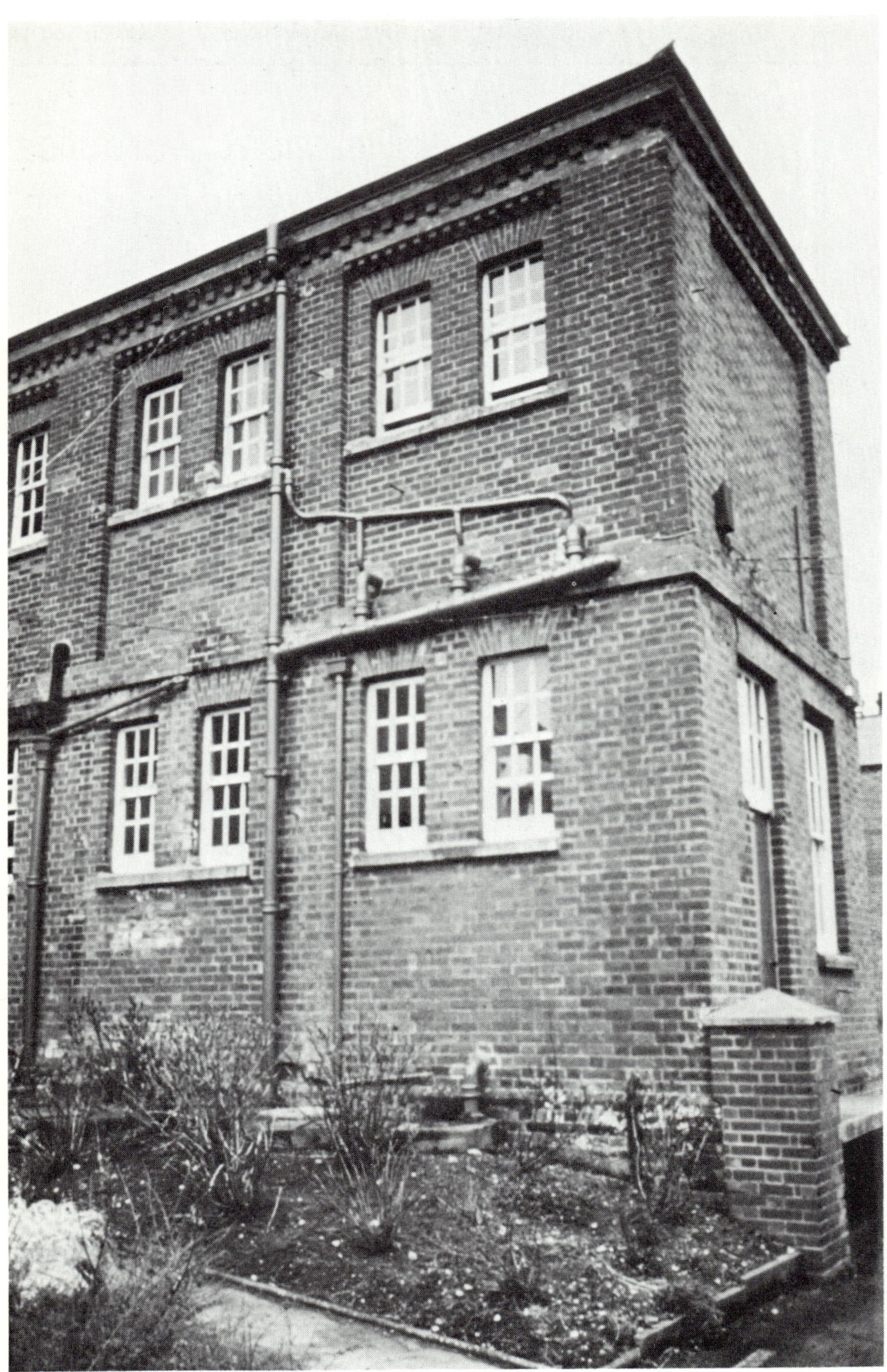

Fig. 6.1 Example of traditional external stacks and vents

work required, often with an unsightly effect on the face of a building. This method of control was not only very expensive, but also unsuitable for certain types of buildings such as high-rise blocks of flats and deep planned factories or hospitals.

(b) Limiting the height of stacks depending upon their size and number of appliances can control the air movement, but restricting the type and number of appliances may increase the complexity of the system and total amount of pipework required.

There will be a risk that, if during the life of the building other appliances are added such as dishwasher or washing machine discharging into a sink, the system may become overloaded. This can also be illustrated by assuming that in a twenty-storey block of flats there is one WC per floor on a 150 mm stack, plus the other usual appliances. If the designer wishes to add another WC per floor he will require another stack – or add a ventilation stack.

(c) The use of pressure relief valves and resealing traps. As we are attempting to prevent the unsealing of appliance traps by siphonage this can be obtained by fitting special traps that are specifically designed not to lose their seals under these conditions. However, they cannot be fitted to all appliances such as WCs which have their own integral traps. To allow air movement through a pipework system it is usual to take a stack through the roof into the open air. This may not always be convenient and can lead to complications in the roof construction as well as the risk of water penetration at the joint.

Another way is to fit an air admittance valve in the roof space or above the topmost appliance flood level; this allows air into a system, but not foul air out (see pp. 104–6).

Resealing traps or air admittance valves will not relieve back pressure so an open vent must be used somewhere in the system.

Siphonage

The effect of siphonage is the removal of an appliance trap water seal due to a pressure drop in the pipework system.

There are two types of siphonage, self siphonage and induced siphonage. Self siphonage is where the full bore flow from an appliance draws the trap water seal with it at the end of the discharge. Research has shown that it is most likely to occur in hand wash basins traps not fitted with spray taps, and waste plugs. It is a function of the cross-sectional shape of the appliance and the bore, length and gradient of the waste pipe.

Induced a siphonage is where the pressure within the pipework system falls below atmospheric due to the air movement caused by the discharge of other appliances. This suction will draw the trap seal of appliances connected to the sys-

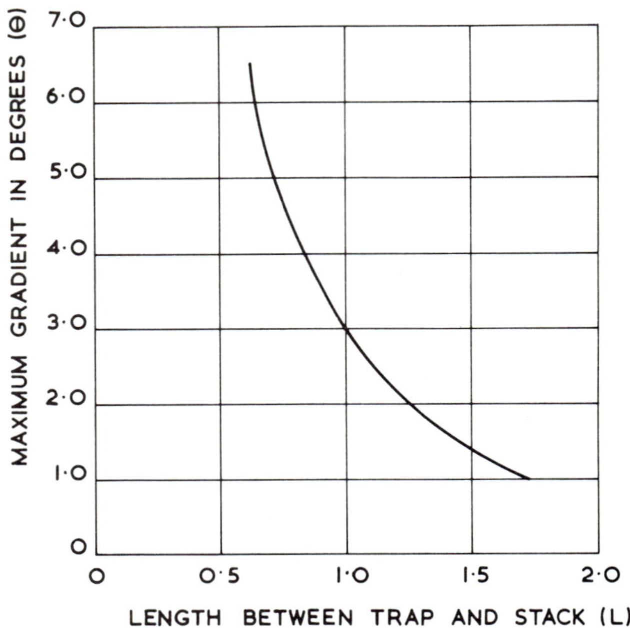

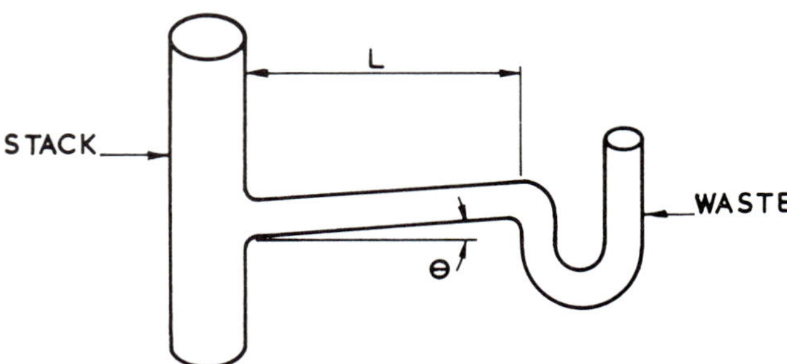

Fig. 6.2 Graph showing British Standard basin waste limits

tem. The method of overcoming induced siphonage is to allow air to move into a system to prevent a drop in air pressure behind the trap; Provide adequate ventilation pipework; and to fit resealing traps to suitable appliances.

Three situations may cause induced siphonage.

(a) A horizontal drain flowing at sufficient depth to cover a branch entry from another appliance will cause the air in the incoming branch to be drawn into the flow with the consequent effect of producing a slight drop in pressure

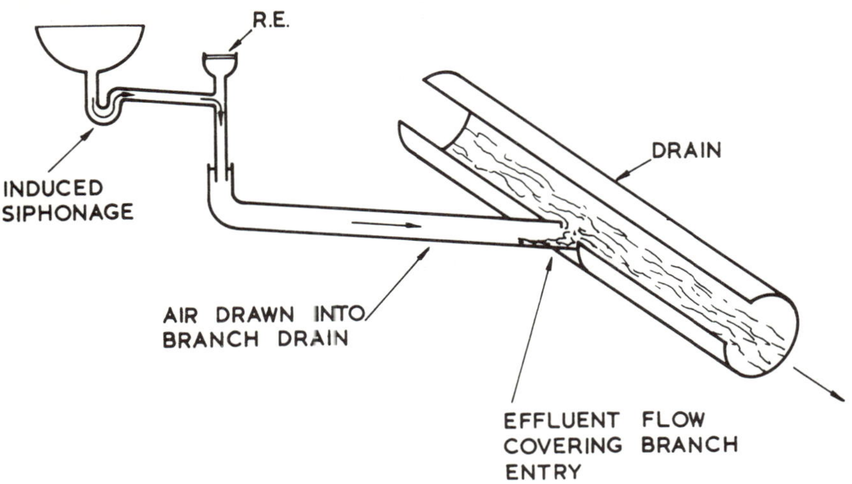

Fig. 6.3 Induced siphonage in branches

within the branch and induced siphonage of the trap. To overcome this, the depth of flow in the main drain should be controlled by size, gradient or by limiting the number of appliances. A branch end vent or air admittance valve could also be used and resealing traps fitted where appropriate.

(b) When effluent discharges into a vertical stack at each floor in a multi-storey building the flow crosses the diameter of the stack, hits the wall on the far side and then flows down the stack as a water film. There is also a central core of air drawn down with the flow of water. Air pressure at the top of the stack falls below atmospheric depending upon the number of appliances discharging and on the diameter of the stack. The flow down the stack is due to the force of gravity, but it does not continue to accelerate. There is a terminal distance down a stack from the point of discharge where the frictional drag of the walls of the stack slow down the acceleration of the water film to a constant speed.

(c) The wind blowing across the top of a stack can cause induced siphonage of the appliances on the top few floors. It can occur in areas of the country such as on the coast or high ground, or if the stack terminates near the edge or corner of a flat-roofed building or level with the top of a parapet.

Back pressure

Back pressure can occur in a drainage system if the air drawn into the pipework by the discharge of appliances is prevented from escaping to atmosphere. This will occur at the base of a stack (see Fig. 6.4); the smaller the bend the greater the effect. A large radius bend, or preferably two 45° bends in combination, should be used.

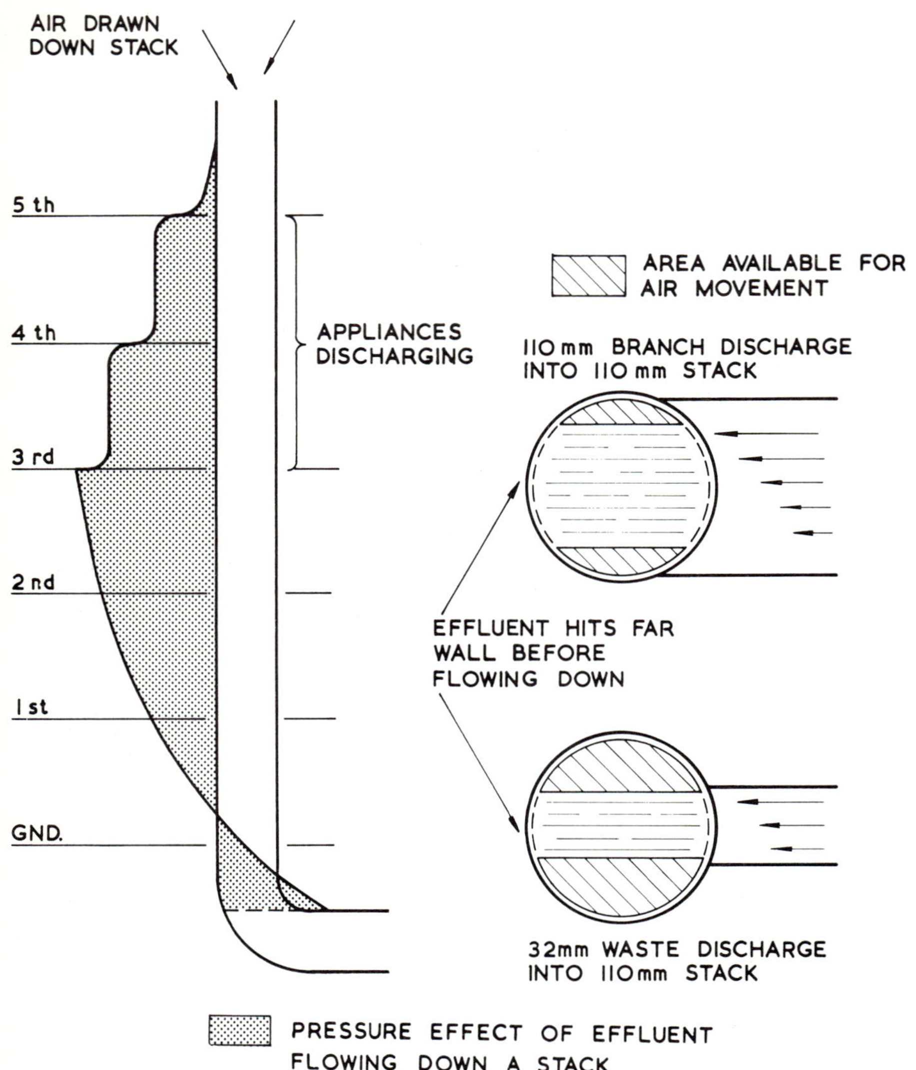

Fig. 6.4 Pressure effects of effluent flowing down a stack

Positive pressure in a vertical stack can also be caused by a build up of detergent foam or bacterial gel, preventing the free movement of air. The provision of a vent at the base of a stack will usually relieve back pressure, but not if the pressure is caused by foam or gel, as the vent connection to the stack may also be blocked.

Offsets in a vertical stack below the topmost appliance can also cause back pressure and venting may be required. Offsets above the topmost appliance have a negligible effect on the flow of air through the system.

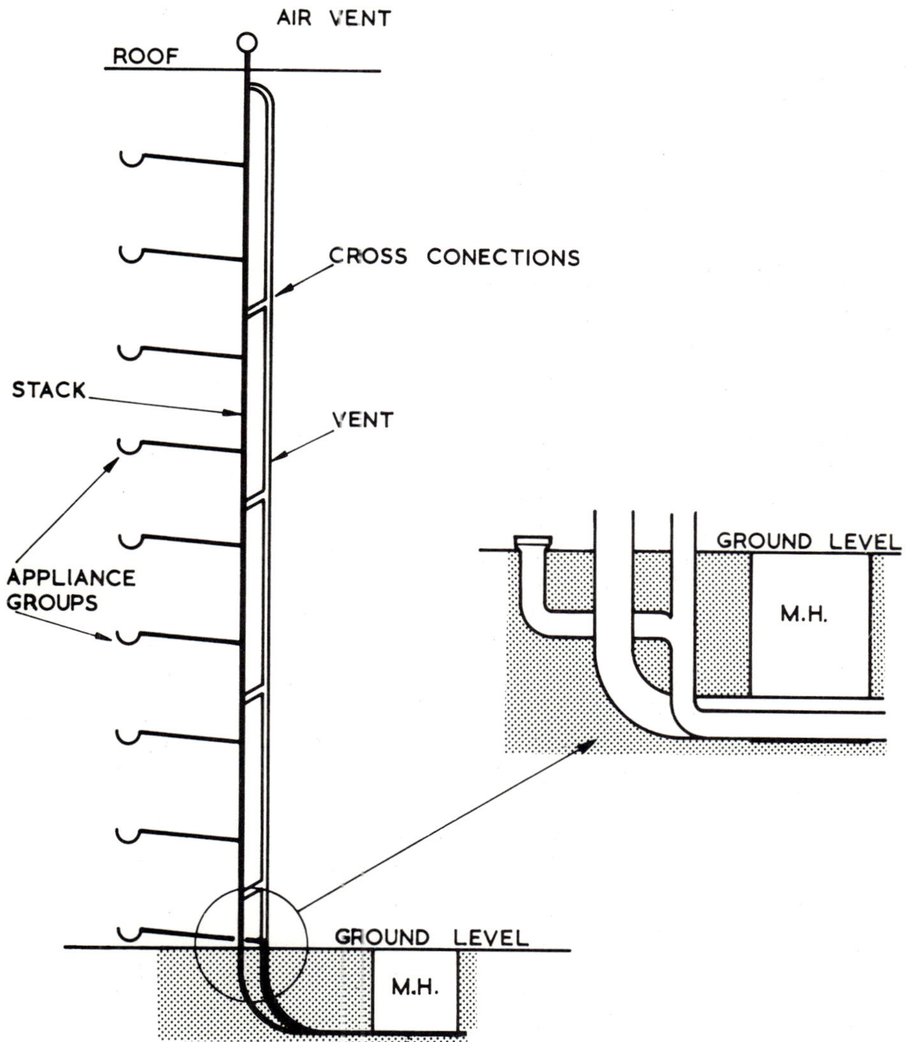

Fig. 6.5 Method of connecting ground floor appliances to the vent stack to obviate back pressure effects

Back pressure can occur in a horizontal system either above or below ground due to a number of practical causes, but fundamentally they are usually caused by a restriction to the free flow of effluent within the system.

If a horizontal pipe is partially blocked a back pressure will develop above the point of the blockage every time an appliance is discharged. Similarly, if a drain is surcharged or has a defective interceptor inadequately vented back pressure will develop.

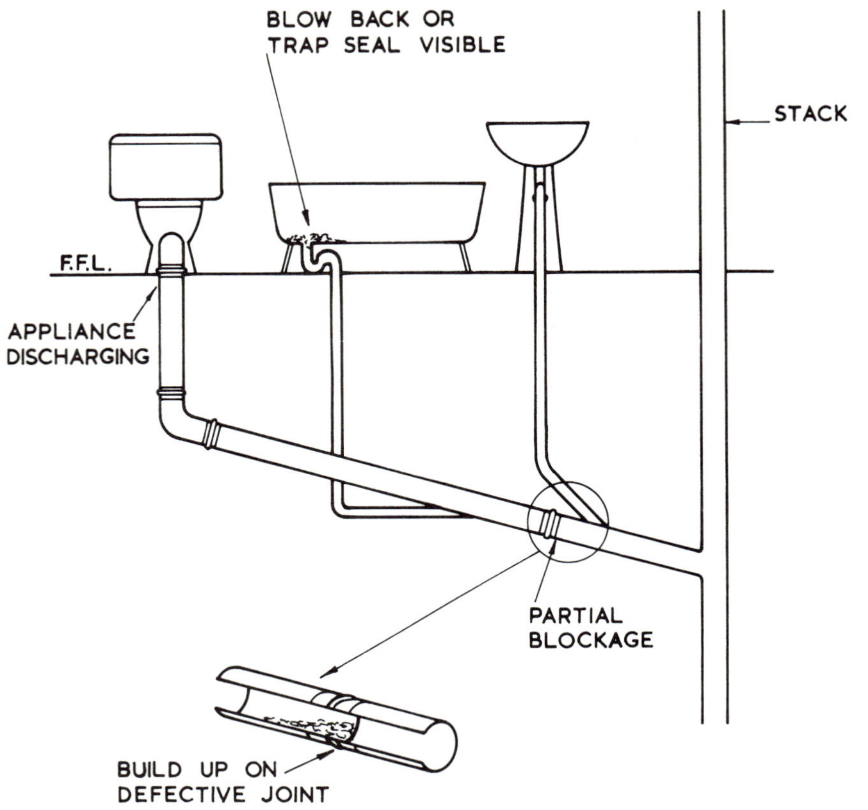

Fig. 6.6 Back pressure in horizontal systems

Consequently, if back pressure – observed by the blowing back of effluent into an appliance, the slow raising of the contents of a trap seal into an appliance or the slow discharge of an appliance – is apparent it is likely that an incipient blockage is developing.

A full blockage prevents the discharge of effluent and blow back can be violent in up-stream appliances.

To prevent overloading a system and causing siphonage and back pressure effects, a knowledge of the likely hydraulic peformance of the system is essential. We therefore require to know how many appliances can be discharged into a system of a given size and gradient, or inversely, for a given number of appliances, what must be the size and gradient of the pipework and what ventilation, if any, must be provided.

User factors

It would obviously be wasteful to design a drainage system on the assumption that all the sanitary appliances connected to the system would be discharged at the same instant in time. What is necessary is an estimate of the probable peak flow load related to the time of day for the various sections of the system. This must take into account that each type of appliance – bath, basin, sink, etc. – will be used at a different time and with differing time intervals between use. They also have different flow characteristics in terms of quantity and rate of discharge.

Observation will show that there is a morning peak and evening peak and on weekends a lunch time smaller peak, and that if the WC is situated in the bathroom it is unlikely to be used at the same time as the bath or basin. In schools and factories the peak use will be in breaks between lessons and shifts and at meal times, while in offices there is a peak in the evening before staff leave for home.

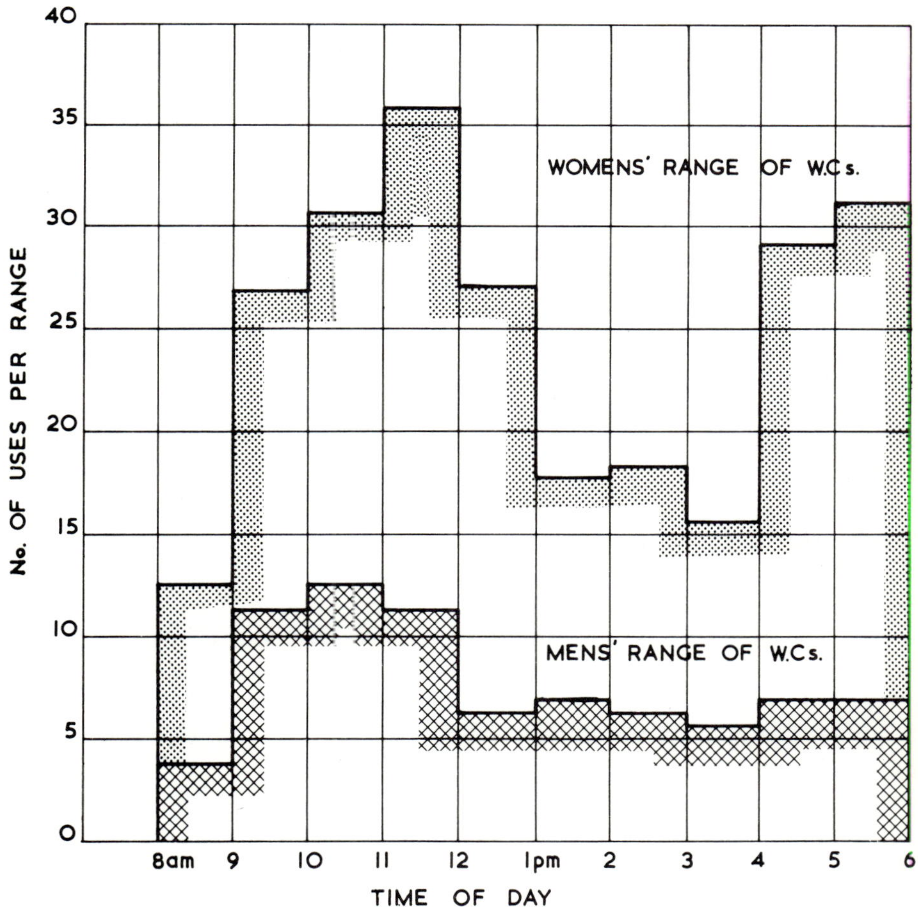

Fig. 6.7 Pattern of use of WCs in an office building

Domestically there is also a day factor which changes the pattern of use. Bath night is still traditionally Friday or Saturday, but as more bath showers are fitted this will affect the flow.

Even favourite television programmes will have an effect, particularly in high rise blocks of flats. Wash days obviously have an effect on the amount of effluent discharged.

As drainage systems are usually installed for the life of the building it is important to allow for change in user pattern.

There has been a general increase in the amount of water used per head of population over the past twenty years, but this may not continue as more dual flush cisterns and showers are installed.

Depth of flow

Because of the various user factors outlined above we must therefore allow for fluctuations in flow in a drainage system, and we must also allow some space for the free movement of air both in horizontal and vertical systems.

The flow capacity for vertical stacks taking the discharge from appliances is usually fixed at about 0.25 full flow – larger flows will result in plugs of falling water and waste forming, giving rise to uncontrollable pressure fluctuations.

Horizontal drains and branches can be designed to flow between 0.5 and 0.75 capacity, but as they do not usually have continuous flow it is difficult to decide where this depth can be measured.

Surface water stacks, drains and branches can be designed to flow full bore although this may lead to gutters overflowing on occasions.

If ponding can be tolerated on a flat roof and sealed manholes are used 110 mm stacks and drains can be used throughout a system (see Ch. 3, p. 32 and Ch. 8, p. 123).

The depth of flow and velocity in a horizontal foul drainage system is also related to the roughness of the pipework material, the shape and quality of the fittings and manhole pipework, and the workmanship and standard of the joints between fittings.

The discharge from a single appliance such as a WC leaves the pan trap at a flow rate of about 2.3 l/s ec., taking only 5 seconds to discharge 9.0 litres. As soon as it enters a horizontal branch the velocity drops proportional to the length of the drain and the effluent extends out, until only a trickle is left along the invert.

The solids are left somewhere on the pipe invert – usually at a joint, bend or junction, and will only be moved on again by the leading edge of the next flush. When discussing velocity and self cleansing flow one should consider where in a system this flow and velocity are to be measured. Only when intermittent flow becomes continuous flow is the velocity relevant.

Pipe sizing

The standard method of pipe sizing currently used in Codes of Practice is based upon a 'discharge unit' value given to appliances or groups of appliances. It is a factor so chosen that the relative load-producing values of the sanitary appliances can be expressed as multiples of that factor. The discharge unit value (DUV) of an appliance depends therefore on the frequency, rate and duration of the use of the appliance.

Research and observations have shown that these factors vary roughly between building types – domestic, public or intense use, and frequency of use classifications are given which alter the DUV of an appliance. The designer must therefore select the appropriate classification related to his assumption of the possible peak frequency of use of the appliances.

Table 6.1 Discharge unit values for some appliances
Frequency between uses: 250 on average for automatic washing machines; 75 domestic bath; 30 hospital or hotel bath; 20 peak domestic; 10 peak commercial; 5 congested, schools, public toilets, exhibitions, etc.

Time interval (min.)	*WC*	*Basin*	*Bath*	*Washing machine*	*Sink*	*Urinal*	*Appliance group*
250	—	—	—	4	—	—	
75	—	—	7	—	—	—	
30	—	—	18	—	—	—	14
20	7	1	—	—	6	0.3	
10	14	3	—	—	14	—	
5	28	6	—	—	27	—	

From Table 6.1 the total DUV can be calculated for any pipework system by simply totalling the number of appliances and adding their DUV together.

The discharge method of design is based upon the hydraulic loading a stack, branch or drain can carry, but it does not give guidance on the venting requirements.

As the size of a discharge stack increases with an increase in the number of appliances the size of the ventilation stack will also increase, and in certain circumstances this may lead to an oversizing of the system.

It is preferable to slightly oversize pipework rather than risk undersizing it as the added cost is usually small. The cost of a drainage system is the cost of installation, excavation and back filling; material costs are usually low, except in specialist materials.

Design process: vertical stacks

The DUV for all the appliances discharging into the stack should be added together. If an appliance is not listed in Table 6.6 an allowance should be made based upon the designer's judgment; a guide is to relate it to a similar appliance.

When the stack also takes continuous flow from equipment some estimate must be made and a DUV given to the discharge. It is however often the case that equipment flows are very low (similar to a shower) and can be discounted.

Table 6.2 Maximum discharge units for stacks

Stack diameter (*mm*)	*Stack capacity* (*l/sec.*)	*No. of discharge units*
75	3.50	200
110	7.00	750
150	22.50	5500

Table 6.3 Maximum discharge units for horizontal branches in stacks

Branch diameter (*mm*)	*Gradient*	*Discharge units*
50	1 in 50	10
	1 in 25	26
75	1 in 100	40
	1 in 50	100
	1 in 25	230
100	1 in 100	230
	1 in 50	430
	1 in 25	1050
150	1 in 100	2000
	1 in 50	3500
	1 in 25	7500

The appropriate stack and branch sizes can be chosen.

Note: Size in many instances is dictated by the outlet of the appliance, or the recommended trap size, as at no time can a pipe that is connected to an outlet from an appliance be less than the diameter of the outlet.

Design Process: horizontal drains flowing continuously

The carrying capacity of a horizontal drain relates directly to the roughness of the material. The roughness is therefore given a factor (k) and is shown in Table 6.4 for the recommended materials.

It is often argued that all pipes develop a film coating, the invert reducing the roughness all to the same factor; but this has not been satisfactorily substantiated.

The carrying capacity in l/sec. is not the only criterion in designing a hori-

Table 6.4 Capacities and discharge unit values for 110 and 150 mm drains for two materials flowing 0.75 full

Drain diameter (mm)	*Gradient*	*Clayware (k = 0.15)*		*PVC (k = 0.003)*	
		Quantity l/sec.	*DUV*	*Quantity l/sec.*	*DUV*
110 (4″)	1 in 50	9.0	1400	11.0	1900
	1 in 100	6.0	630	7.0	830
150 (6″)	1 in 50	28.0	8900	31.0	10800
	1 in 100	19.0	4900	22.0	6200
	1 in 150	16.0	3700	18.0	4500
	1 in 250	12.0	2200	14.0	2900

zontal drainage system, the velocity is also considered important; a general historical recommendation of 2.5 ft/sec. (0.75 m/sec.) is often quoted.

A recent extensive survey has, however, indicated that much lower velocities are acceptable and it is more important to ensure that the quality of the drain is good and that the frequency and quantity of the discharge in relation to the depth of the flow is adequate.

When a branch drain with intermittent flow is infrequently used there is a tendency for deposits to be left on the invert. These may stick if allowed to dry out, in particular if the solid content of the effluent is high. By increasing the water content of the effluent and the frequency of the discharges, the drain will be kept cleaner.

It is a misconception that to increase the size of a drain will reduce the risk of blockages. The exact opposite is the case, for by increasing the size the velocity is reduced and the water is spread over a greater wall surface of the pipe, thereby lowering the depth of flow.

The best hydraulic method to prevent blockages developing is to have a continuous flow at about 0.75 full depth.

Table 6.5 Roughness factors (*k*). Recommended materials in normal condition

Pipework material	*Roughness factor (k) normal condition*
PVC and glass	0.003
Spun iron	0.06
Clayware	0.15

The maximum number of DUV that can be loaded on to a given drain, taken for various gradients and roughness factors, are shown in Table 6.5. It is assumed that pipework and the installation for new works will be of **normal** quality, but for extensions to existing buildings the designs may be discharging into an old, existing system. In this case a TV survey may be required to ascer-

Table 6.6 Quantities and velocities for full bore flow

Pipe Diameter (mm)	*Gradient*	*PVC and glass (k = 0.003)*		*Claywork (k = 0.15)*	
		V (m/sec.)	*Q (l/sec.)*	*V (m/sec.)*	*Q (l/sec.)*
110	1 in 50	1.60	13.0	1.40	11.0
	1 in 100	1.10	8.0	0.90	7.0
150	1 in 50	2.0	35.0	1.70	31.0
	1 in 100	1.40	25.0	1.20	21.5
229	1 in 100	2.50	70.0	1.55	63.0
	1 in 150	1.80	60.0	1.20	50.0
	1 in 200	1.20	50.0	1.10	44.0
	1 in 250	1.05	45.0	1.0	39.0
305	1 in 150	1.90	150.0	1.50	110.0
	1 in 200	1.45	120.0	1.30	94.0
	1 in 250	1.35	105.0	1.15	84.0

Table 6.7 Factors for reducing depth of flow

Depth of flow	*V (m/sec.)*	*Q (l/sec.)*
0.5	1.0	0.5
0.75	1.15	0.9

tain the condition of the old system. A hydraulic test should also be applied and the system cleared of any deposit.

If the condition of the system is less than normal or orther materials have been used, k factors can be taken from the Hydraulics Research Station papers on the design of channels and pipes.

Example of hydraulic design using discharge units

A forty-storey office block has four flats in the top storeys. All the appliances discharge into one vertical stack and thereby into one underground drain. Assuming there are two WCs and two basins per office floor and one WC basin, bath, sink and washing machine per flat, find the size of the stack and the drain size, gradient and material.

From Table 6.1 we can ascertain the DUV for the appliances.

Flats: domestic use.

4 WCs	× 7 DU	= 28
4 basins	× 1 ″	= 4
4 baths	× 7 ″	= 28
4 washing machines	× 4 ″	= 16
		76

Office: peak commercial.

36 WCs	× 28 DU	=	1080
36 basins	× 6″	=	216
	Total		1372

From Table 6.2 the DU total for the stack is greater than that allowed for a 110 mm pipe but well below that allowed for a 150 mm stack. We must therefore design to the 150 mm stack, and as the underground drain cannot be smaller than the incoming stack (see p. 32), from Table 6.4 we can select a clayware drain (k–0.15) at a minimum gradient of 1 in 250.

Continuous flow

Although the usual flow in an underground drainage system is intermittent, continuous flow may occur under certain circumstances.

It certainly will occur in surface water drains as long as the rain is falling, and if land drains discharge via mud sumps into this system it may occur for a considerably longer period, possibly permanently. It may also occur in foul water systems if ground water enters through a defective pipe or joint; and where the system is combined it will occur again. In these cases the flow in the drain should be calculated from the run-off figures available. It is usual to design for a rainfall of 75 mm/hour occurring for a 5-minute period, which, from statistics, may occur once in 4 years or for 20 minutes once in 50 years.

It is worth remembering that 1 mm of rainfall on 1 m^2 of area is 1 litre in quantity.

When designing surface water and roof drainage systems it is advisable to consult any local meteorological information as conditions vary, particularly in coastal areas. Charts and tables for the Hydraulic Design of Storm-drains, Sewers and Pipe lines are available from the Hydraulics Research Station and relate the capacity and velocity of flow to the diameter, gradient and roughness of the pipework.

It is at the discretion of the designer to choose the factors relating to his system, but he must remember that the cost of an underground system is the price of excavation and back filling. It is therefore advisable to keep the gradient as flat as possible.

Advantage should be taken of the contours of the ground, particularly if it is possible to discharge surface water to a stream or water course – usually down hill. Acceptable gradients are 1 in 100, or 1 in 150, for a 110 mm pipe and 1 in 150, or 1 in 200 for a 150 mm pipe. Flatter than this may give installation problems and lead to backfalls which, although not hydraulically unacceptable, can lead to sedimentation in the inverts of the backfalls.

Table 6.8 Discharge unit valves and capacities for horizontal drains flowing 0.75 full bore

Drain diameter (mm)	*Gradient*	*PVC and glass*		*Clayware*	
		DUV	*0.75 flow (l/sec.)*	*DUV*	*0.75 flow (l/sec.)*
100	1 : 60	1 600	12.0	1 100	10.0
	1 : 100	880	7.0	630	6.0
150	1 : 60	9 600	29.0	8 000	25.0
	1 : 100	6 200	22.0	4 900	19.0
	1 : 150	4 500	18.0	3 700	16.0
	1 : 250	2 900	14.0	2 200	12.0
229	1 : 100	21 000	63.0	16 000	57.0
(225 Clay)	1 : 150	16 000	55.0	12 000	47.0
(250 PVC)	1 : 200	12 500	45.0	9 500	39.0
	1 : 250	10 500	40.0	8 000	35.0
305	1 : 150	50 000	125.0	37 000	100.0
(300 Clay)	1 : 200	40 000	110.0	30 000	85.0
	1 : 250	30 000	100.0	23 000	75.0

Note: It is assumed that for sizes above 150 mm continuous flow is being experienced.

Table 6.9 Main drain sizing by discharge unit valves

Drain point	*DUV totals*	*Table DUV (Max.)*	*Gradients*		*Remarks*
			Clay	*PVC*	
(1)	2000	2200	1 : 250		Little spare capacity
		2900		1 : 250	
(2)	3350	3700	1 : 150		Some spare capacity
		4500		1 : 150	
(3)	4700	4900	1 : 100		Some spare capacity
		4500		1 : 150	No spare capacity
(4)	6050	8000	1 : 60		
		6200		1 : 100	Little spare capacity
(5)	8760	8000	1 : 60		Overloaded
		9600		1 : 60	

To design an underground foul drainage system where continuous flow may be experienced the values shown in Table 6.8 should be used. It is a matter of adding together all the stack and branch drain DUV flows into the main drain and sizing accordingly, at the same time choosing the gradient and material. The gradient will depend upon the inverts available.

Example: If we therefore take the design shown in Fig. 6.8 of five stacks discharging each 1350 DUVs into a main drain, the sizes and gradients for a 150 mm pipe are shown accordingly (Table 6.9).

Without the site sloped in the direction of the drain a gradient of 1 in 60 would be uneconomical and a 229 mm drain at a gradient of 1 in 250 would be used either in clayware or PVC.

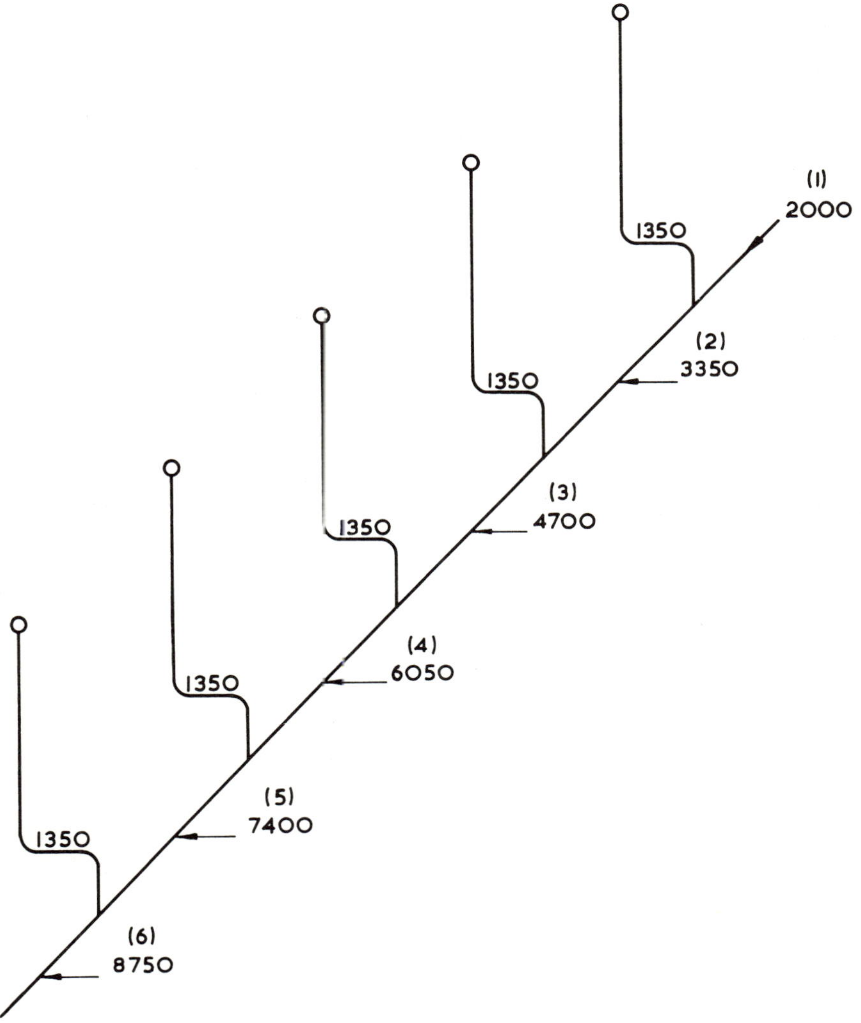

Fig. 6.8 Drain sizing by discharge unit values

Chapter 7

Ventilation

Introduction

The provision of external, above-ground discharge pipework systems with attached ventilation pipework of approximately the same diameter as the discharge pipe was traditionally accepted until about 1948 when changes in regulations and building design practices brought the pipework within the building envelope.

With the growth in popularity of high-rise flats and office blocks it became impractical to use this traditional method of vent pipework and a new system of drainage was developed where all the pipework is contained within internal ducts.

It was also realized that to provide virtually a double system of pipework – discharge pipe and vent pipe – was expensive in material, labour and space, consequently research was carried out at the Building Research Station and on selected sites to investigate the hydraulics and pneumatics of these systems with the objective of improving them by reducing the amount of pipework until then considered necessary, without lowering their performance standards.

Research was firstly concentrated on pipework systems for dwellings up to twelve storeys in height using a 110 mm single stack system. This area of study was later enlarged to consider dwellings up to twenty-five storeys in height and office blocks using 150 mm stacks in cast iron, then the traditionally accepted material for above-ground systems.

This research showed that the 110 mm and 150 mm systems were adequate for many types of buildings, but there was also a theoretical hydraulic requirement for a 5-inch (125 mm) single stack system. This size, however, did not become popular with the majority of pipework manufacturers who were at that time attempting to rationalize their manufacturing capacity, or stockists who did not want to add an extra completely new range of pipes and fittings to their already large stocks. It failed therefore for purely commercial reasons, particularly as the cost of delivery and installation was little more than for the 150 mm size.

Further research both in the laboratory and on site has been undertaken to investigate the venting requirements for office systems and also those used in

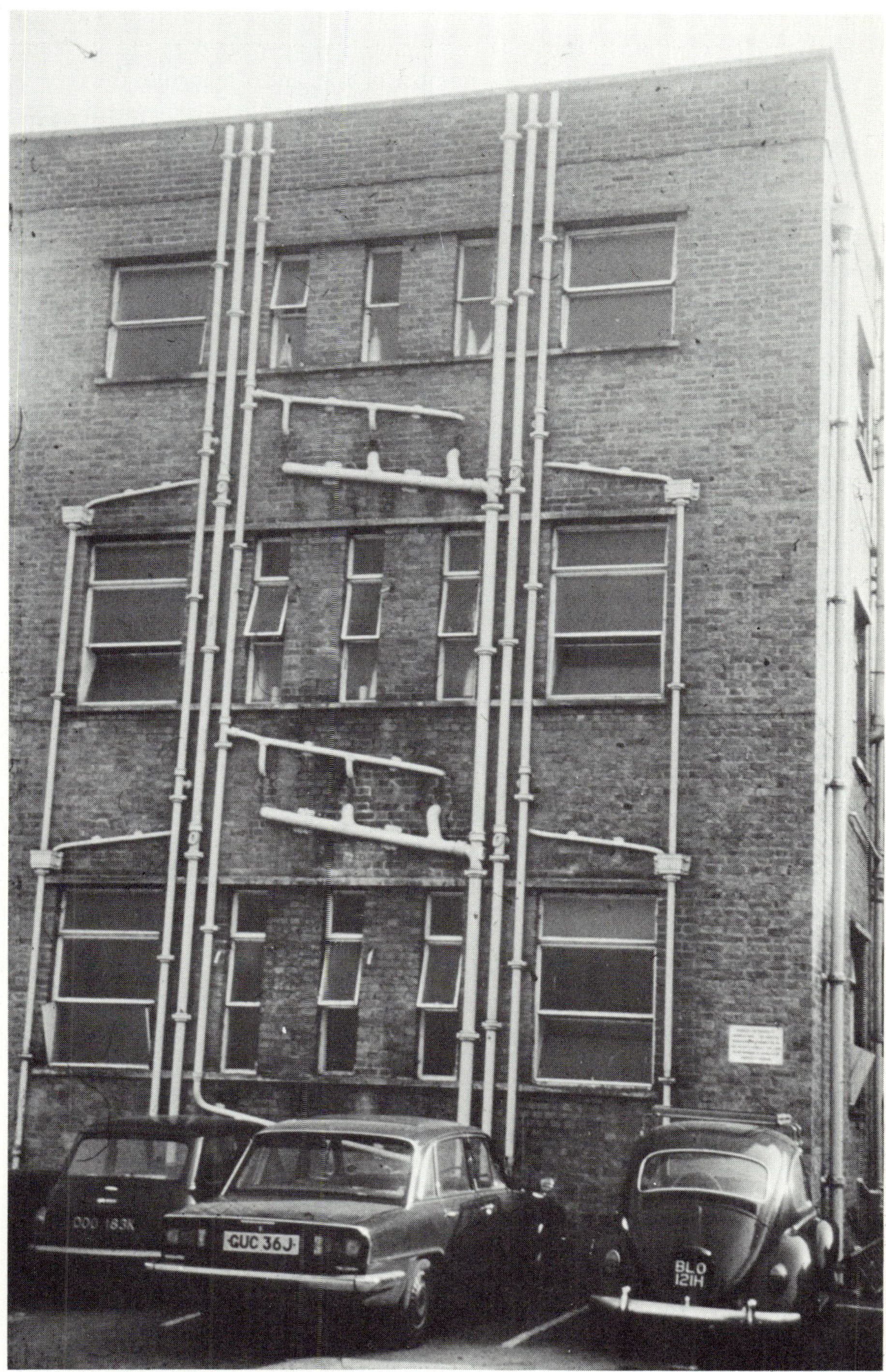

Fig. 7.1 Traditional external system

hospitals. It was discovered that in many cases there is no need to provide any ventilation pipework at all, adequate ventilation being provided by the open end of the discharge stack; but where the number of appliances related to the type of usage, and height of the building suggests that a single stack system is inappropriate, some ventilation will be required. It will also be required where horizontal branches take the flow from a large number of appliances likely to be discharged at the same time, such as in public buildings or schools, or where the design of the building necessitates the use of offsets or bends in the discharge pipework system.

Underground systems

The ventilation of the underground drainage system is usually via the building discharge stacks, but in many old buildings this is effectively prevented by the use of interceptor traps. This device prevents the free flow of air within the system and required a fresh air inlet valve containing a one-way mica flap fitted adjacent to the manhole containing the interceptor.

These interceptors are known causes of drain blockages and should not be fitted in new works on combined or foul drainage systems, but may be necessary where a surface water drain discharges into a foul or combined drain to prevent sewer gases from venting through the rainwater gutters or down pipes.

Objectives

The reason for ventilating the drainage system is to keep the air pressure within the pipework at or near atmospheric and to prevent rapid pressure fluctuations occurring due to the discharge of appliances, or the movement of effluents which may adversely affect the appliance trap water seals, or creates unacceptable noise.

Pressure fluctuations can be negative, causing suction and thereby draw trap seals allowing foul air into the building, or positive when back pressure may blow back foul air through the water seals. Both positive and negative pressure changes can cause unacceptable noise.

The design of the total drainage system including any ventilation pipework must limit these pressure changes so that they do not exceed ± 38 mm water gauge or that the appliance traps retain at least 25 mm water seal.

As well as pressure fluctuations developed by the flow of effluent within the pipework they can also be caused by the effect of wind blowing across the top of an open stack or vent terminal, particularly when they are sited in the vicinity of parapets or corners of buildings.

The provision of ventilation pipework will not prevent seal losses due to wind effects, and terminal positions may have to be moved or air admittance valves fitted.

Regulations

Although drain gases are not generally pathogenic they can be obnoxious and therefore terminals must not be positioned where the release of such gases can pass into a building.

The Building Regulations are specific in their requirements and any pipe not being a drain and open to the external air at the highest point which ventilates a drainage system must be carried up to a height of not less than 900 mm above the head of any window or opening into a building such as a roof light, and at a horizontal distance away from such an opening of at least 3.0 m in such a manner as not to become prejudicial to health or a nuisance, and fitted at its topmost end with a durable wire cage or other cover to prevent the entry of objects likely to block the systems or prevent the free movement of air, but such cover must in itself not unduly restrict the flow of air.

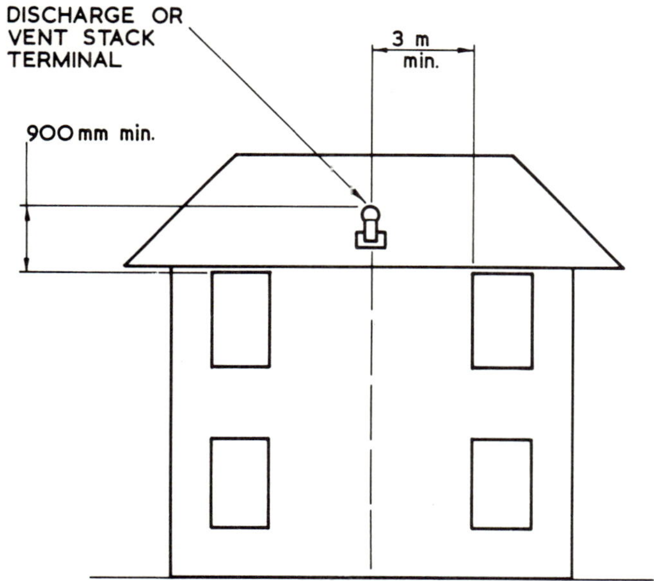

Fig. 7.2 Mandatory recommendations for vent terminals

Installation

Research has shown that a very small diameter vent pipe will allow sufficient air movement throughout a drainage system to prevent pressure fluctuations that may be detrimental to the water seals in appliance traps, and that the length of the vent and the number of bends and offsets does not unduly reduce the flow of air throughout the system, although they should preferably be of large radius.

It has been found that a 25 mm vent pipe is adequate for many branch ventilation systems, but if the branch is longer than 15 m or contains more than five bends (two bends form one offset) this size should be increased to 32 mm. If there is a possibility of the vent being subjected to flooding it should be increased to 42 or even 50 mm. Practically, a 42 mm vent is the smallest size recommended.

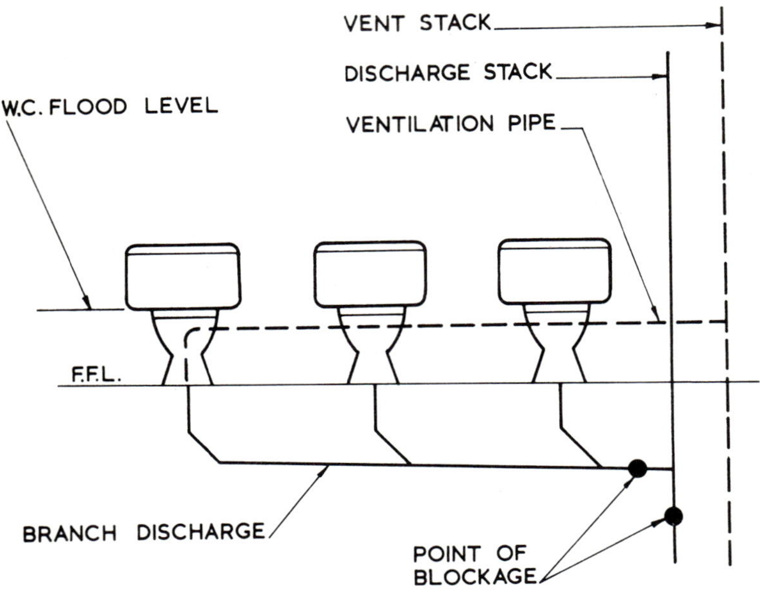

Fig. 7.3 Ventilation pipework liable to flood

The horizontal vent pipe shown in Fig. 7.3 has been hidden behind the WCs and consequently is below their flood level if a blockage develops; it would then fill with effluent before the WCs overflowed. Although the recommended fall back to the discharge pipe is shown it is possible for the bore of the vent pipe to become blocked or at least reduced in diameter due to solids being left in the pipe.

Access into the vent pipe system should always be provided so that if a blockage in this situation occurs it can be cleaned out as part of the maintenance procedure.

It is not recommended under any circumstances to position any horizontal section of a vent pipe below appliance flood level, and all such horizontal vents should always be graded to fall back to a discharge pipe to ensure that it is kept free from water which would otherwise accumulate due to condensation within the system. The only places this rule does not apply are shown in Fig. 7.4(a) where a vent pipe is connected into a discharge pipe above the topmost appliance in the system, and Fig. 7.4 (b) where a loop above flood level of an appliance then falls below floor level and runs back to the vent stack.

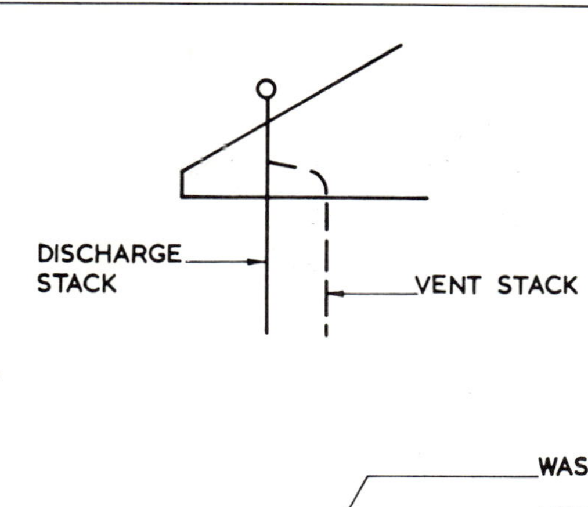

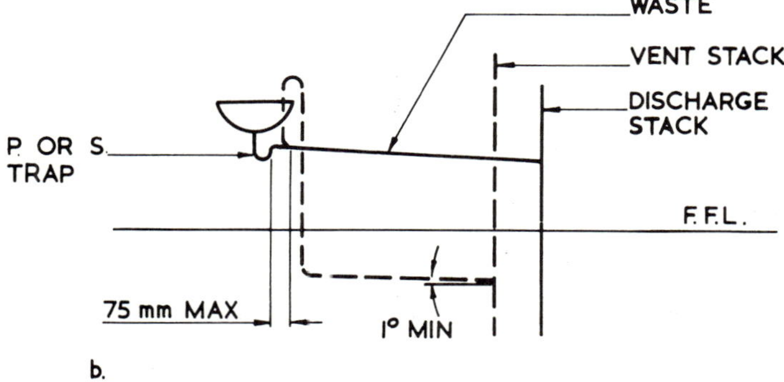

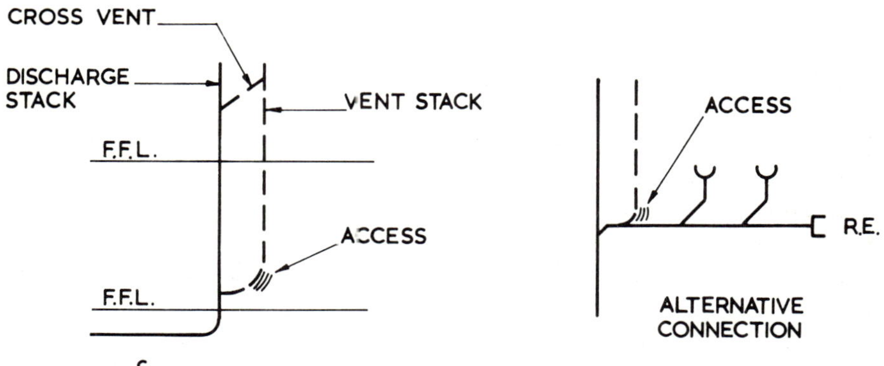

Fig. 7.4 Vent/discharge stack connections

The vent stack must always connect into the discharge stack in the direction of flow (Fig. 7.4c) and should be provided with an access point.

Cast iron vent stacks have been known to collect rust at their base which if not cleaned out at planned intervals may cause a blockage, thereby preventing the free movement of air within the system. It is also not unknown for small birds to find their way into a stack and cause a blockage if the cage is not in position or has partially corroded away.

In certain circumstances the discharge stack may have to be offset or bent; in these cases unacceptable pressure fluctuations may occur and venting should be provided. Only in lightly loaded systems up to three storeys in height will no venting be required, but the bends or offsets must be of large radius, e.g. at least 200 mm. Branches into a stack must not connect on the bend or offset.

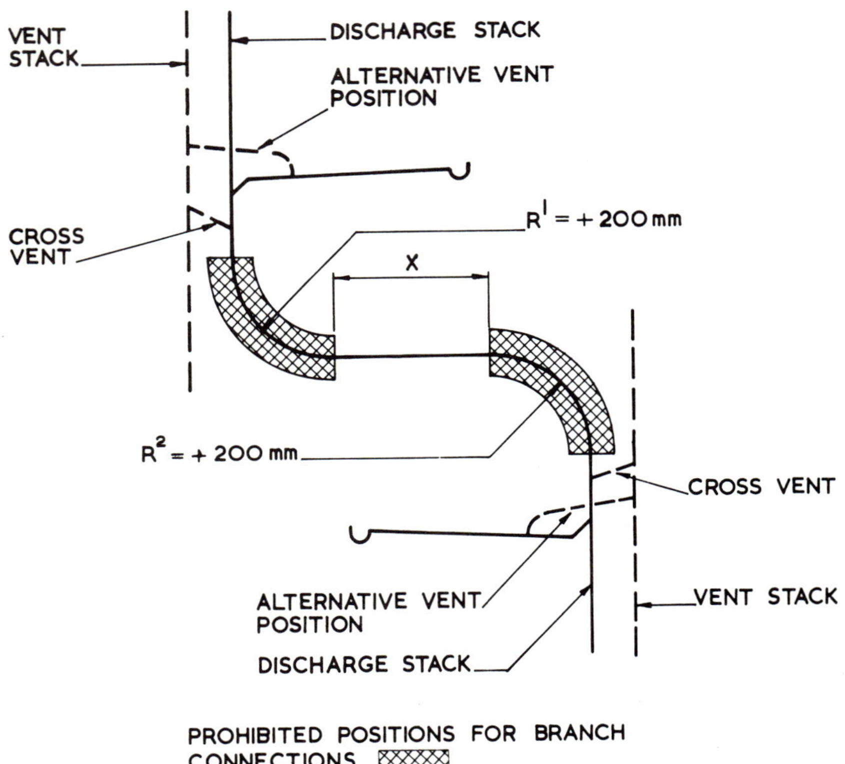

Fig. 7.5 Prohibited positions for branch connections

Cross connections must slope from the vent stack to the discharge stack at an angle of approximately 67½ degrees maximum and the connecting pipe should be the same diameter as the vent stack.

For branch pipes of less than 50 mm in diameter it is preferable to connect the vent stack directly into the branch as close to the appliance trap as possible.

For branch pipes of 75 mm and above the vent cross connection can be made into the top of the branch adjacent to where it joins the discharge stack.

Typical vent/discharge stack arrangements

In certain types of building such as hospitals it may be necessary to combine the wastes from certain appliances, but there is always a possibility with such systems that one appliance when discharging may pull the trap seal of the appliance enjoying the same waste, or create a back pressure that may blow through the seal. If a resealing type trap is not used on the basin a vent should be fitted which will also overcome back pressure and noise.

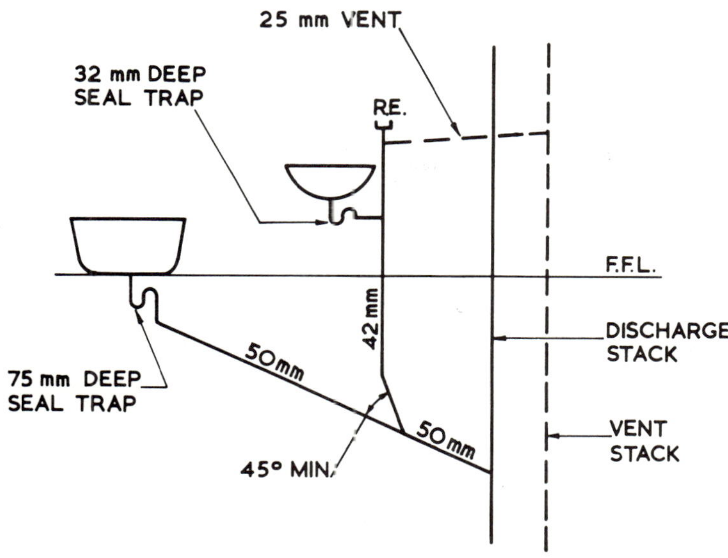

Fig. 7.6 Combined wastes

It is inadvisable to combine the wastes of more than two appliances into a 42 mm common pipe, although this rule does not apply when the appliances are fitted with spray taps or showers, when up to five may be coupled to the same waste. Experience has shown that when combining wastes it is preferable to use 50 mm pipework, although there is a very small increase in material costs.

Washing machines and dish washers

These pieces of equipment usually discharge via a flexible hose and should drain into a trapped standing waste of 42 mm diameter which has an air gap to allow for pressure variations during the discharge period (Fig. 7.7a). If this connection is sealed a 25 mm vent will be required (Fig. 7.7b).

In ground floor positions the waste pipe may discharge above the water level, but below the grating of an external gully when no venting will be required.

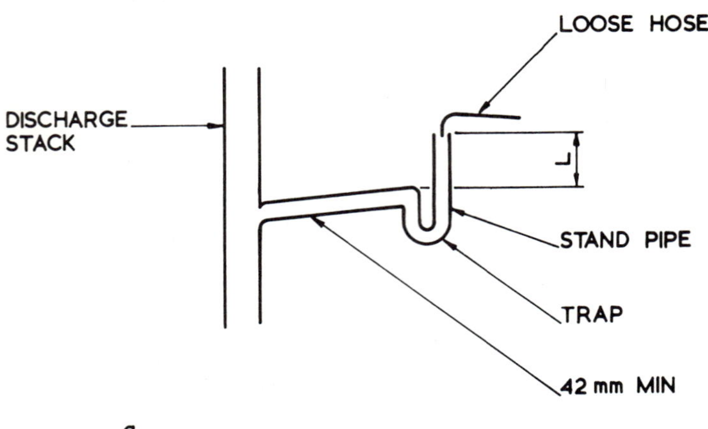

'L' IS DEPENDENT UPON THE MACHINE DESIGN

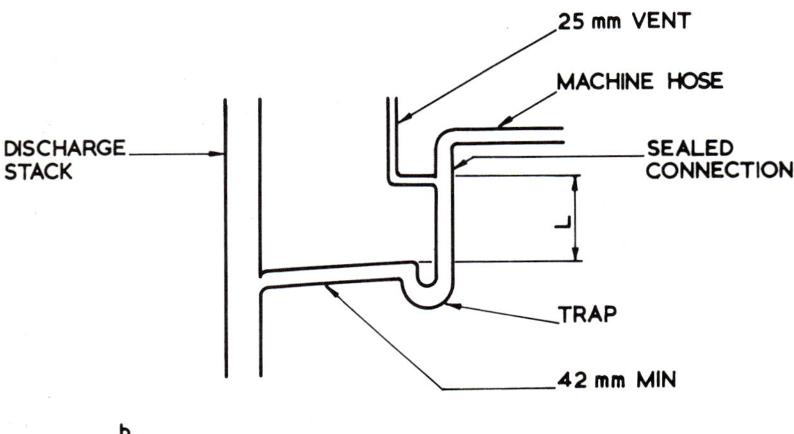

Fig. 7.7 Venting to machine waste

When the machine waste has an air gap there is some risk of internal flooding if the waste becomes blocked, but if the air gap is sealed and no vent provided the machine may self siphon.

Any vent must be taken outside the building.

Range of appliances

Ranges of wash basin wastes will, if not fitted with resealing type traps, require a 25 mm vent pipe, but if spray taps and flush waste outlets are fitted no vent will be necessary for ranges of up to five basins. When the branch waste is less than 4.5 m in length, 'P' or 'S' traps can be used.

Horizontal branches on drains of 75 mm and above are unlikely to flow full bore and therefore should not require venting. Ranges of WCs on branch pipes will only require venting if there are more than two bends in the branch or more than eight WCs in close connection.

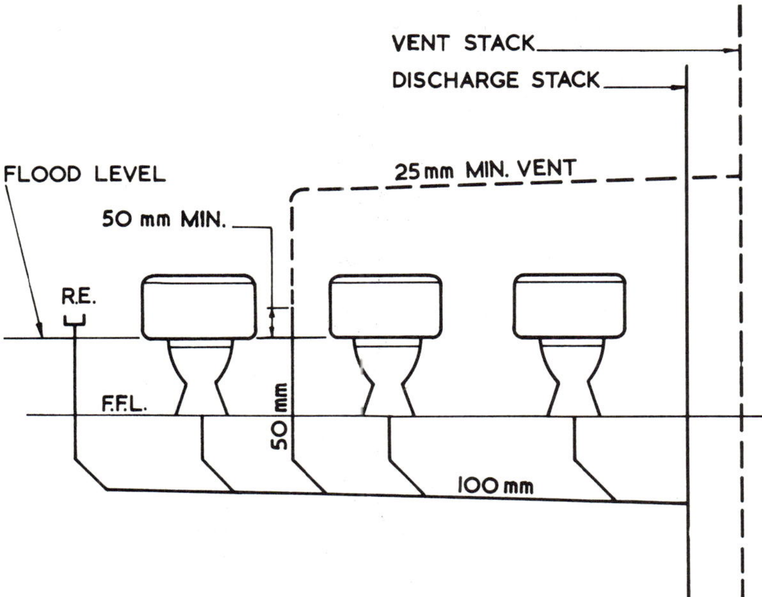

Fig. 7.8 Venting for WC ranges

Direct connections

Direct connections from either a single appliance, or a group of appliances via a stub stack into a horizontal system, should not require venting but should only be contemplated if the drain is adequately ventilated or there may be a possibility of back pressure blowing back through the trap seals or siphonage occurring.

Air admittance valves

It has been the practice in Sweden and other European countries for a number of years to use air admittance valves in place of open stacks to allow air to enter the drainage system, thereby balancing the siphonage effect of appliance discharging. This practice has extended into the United Kingdom, encouraged by the issue of Agrément Certificate (No. 82/977) for the Durgo valve. Its application has appealed to the imagination of designers and planners as well as those persons concerned with the maintenance of roof structures be they pitched or flat.

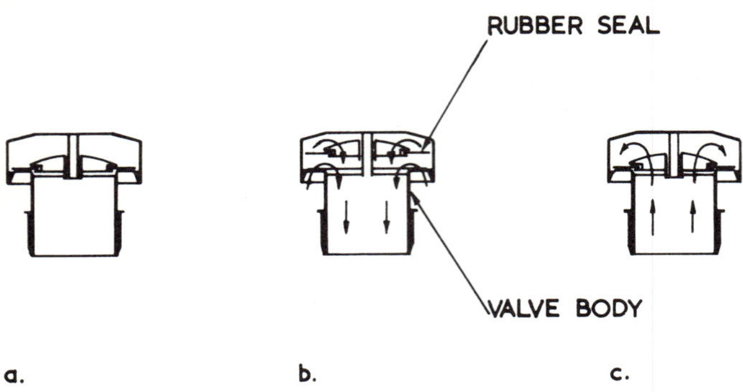

Fig. 7.9 Section through the 'Durgo valve'

Mechanics

Figure 7.9 (a) shows the valve in a closed position with the rubber sealing disk down; the system is at atmospheric pressure. Figure 7.9 (b) shows that when the system is subjected to negative pressure the sealing disk lifts, allowing air to be drawn into the discharge system, thereby effectively preventing trap seal loss by siphonage.

If positive pressure occurs the disk remains closed and is pressed tighter on to the seating, preventing foul air from escaping into the building.

Application

The valve is manufactured in plastic and its spigot is adapted with an ABS sleeve to fit unplasticized PVC soil pipes to BS 5255 for the 50 mm size and BS 4514 for the 75 mm and 110 mm sizes, when connected with adaptors they can be used with other pipework materials.

When the underground drain and foot of the stack bend are of 110 mm diameter sanitary appliances must not be connected to the stack on the lower two floors, or the overall height of the system must be limited to three floors.

When the underground drain and bend at the base of the stack are of 150 mm or more no restrictions are placed on the lower two floors and the valves may be used in buildings up to ten storeys in height.

The valves must be positioned within the drainage system where they will not be subjected to flooding if a blockage occurs and they should be reasonably accessible for maintenance or inspection.

Valves should not be used on stacks where surcharging of the underground drainage system may occur or where there is an interceptor in the system preventing the free flow of air.

They may be used to replace conventional venting arrangements and are particularly useful in horizontal systems where end venting may be considered necessary.

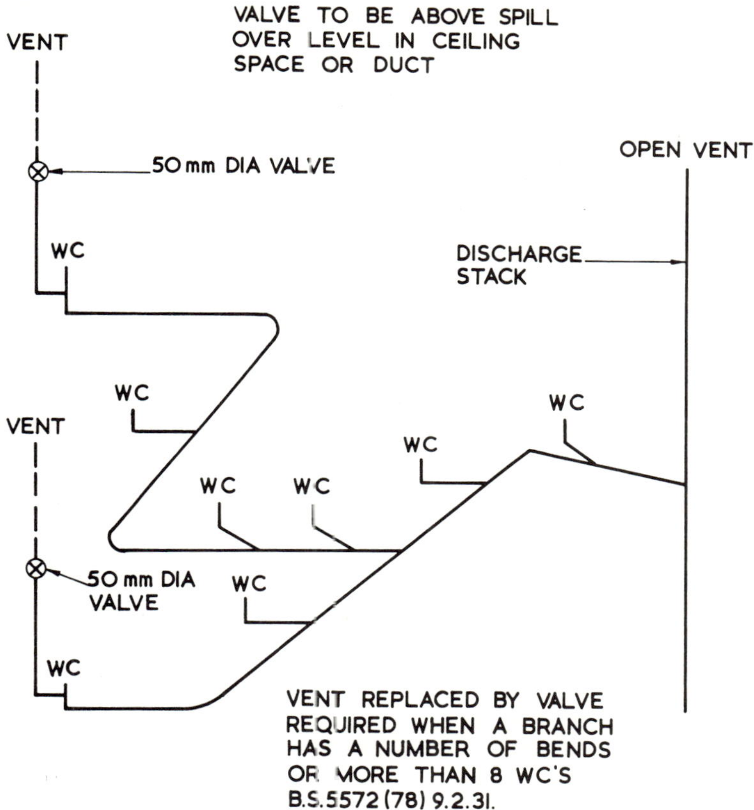

Fig. 7.10 Typical horizontal system using valves

To reduce the effect of back pressures developing there should be one open-ended stack within the network.

Advantages

The main advantage of using an air admittance valve to replace more conventional vent pipework is that by not penetrating the roof structure or waterproof membrane there is no risk of water finding its way into the roof at the penetration.

Pipework penetrating a roof can cause a cold bridge effect, allowing condensation to occur within the structure and related problems of dampness, and in areas of high wind the position of a traditional roof drain terminal may cause siphonage of trap seals. These effects do not occur when the stacks terminated are below the roof finish when a valve is used.

There will also be some cost savings as not only can the roof slate be omitted,

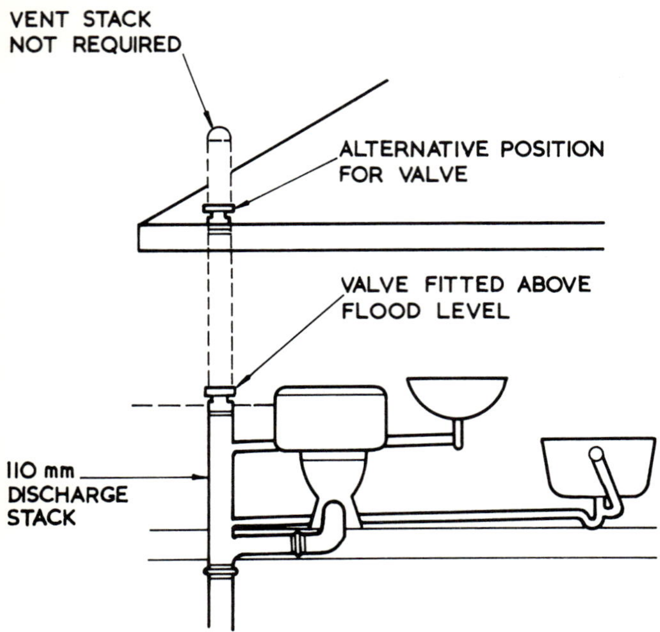

Fig. 7.11 Typical domestic pipework arrangement

but there will be a significant reduction in pipework, well illustrated in the ventilated system using valves.

Venting to office drainage systems

Traditional practice for designing office drainage systems has required that each individual sanitary appliance should be provided with its own vent connection linked to an elaborate network of vent pipes and resulting in nearly doubling the amount of installed pipework. Not only was this expensive and wasteful in materials, but extremely unsightly.

Research and site testing has shown that a much simpler system of vent pipework is adequate, particularly if resealing traps and air admittance valves are used.

Design

When designing a vertical drainage system for an office building it is recommended that two 45 degree bends are used at the base of the stack to reduce the effect of back pressure, and that large radius bends are used in all other situations with adequate access for maintenance purposes in positions where they will not be submerged if flooding occurs.

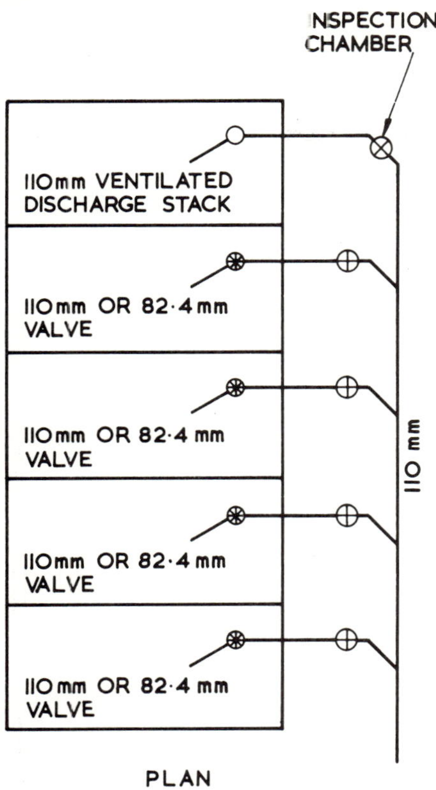

Fig. 7.12 Typical venting provision for terraced dwellings

The flow from various combinations of appliances can be equated as shown in Table 7.1.

In offices or similar buildings up to twenty-four storeys in height with 150 mm discharge stacks vent stacks will only be necessary when the peak usage of the appliances is less than 5 minute intervals, or where there are more than three WCs plus three basins on repetitive floors, or the stacks are offset.

In similar buildings up to four floors in height using a 100 mm discharge stack no vent pipework will be required when there are groups of three WCs plus three basins or less and when the interval between WC usages is 5 minutes or more, or with five WCs plus five basins when this interval is 10 minutes or more, or the stacks are offset. Outside these parameters vent pipework may be required.

Horizontal systems

Long horizontal drainage systems either below ground or slung in an interfloor

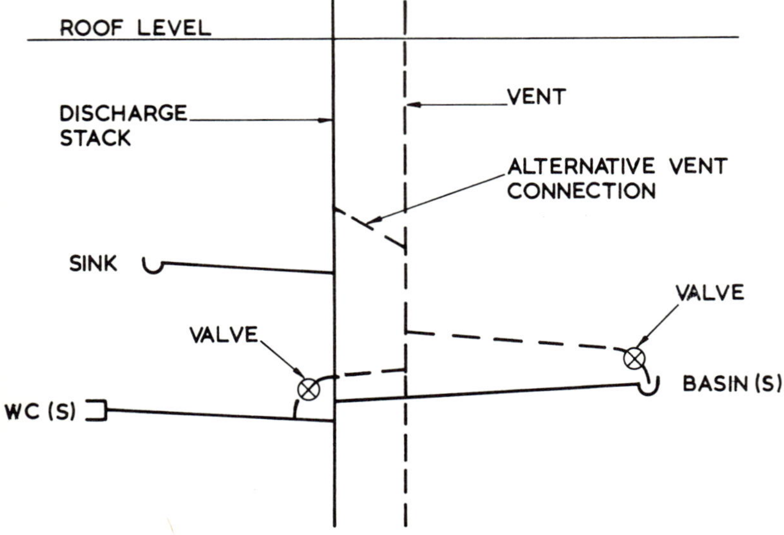

Fig. 7.13 Typical ventilated system replaced by valves

Table 7.1 Appliance groups

WC		*Basin*		*Urinal*		*WC*		*Basin*
2	+	1	+	2	=	2	+	2
2	+	2	+	3	=	3	+	3
3	+	3	+	4	=	4	+	4
4	+	4	+	5	=	5	+	5

zone require some ventilation pipework to balance the air pressure that may develop. In an underground situation this is usually provided by the open discharge stacks, but if air admittance valves are fitted relief ventilation should be provided up stream at the head of the sytem (Fig. 7.12).

Horizontal systems within buildings also require some ventilation and 32 mm or 42 mm end vents should be provided to all main runs. Branch ventilation can be via 25 mm vents.

Chapter 8

Design and installation

Introduction

It has been impossible up to this chapter not to discuss 'design and installation' in relation to the various aspects of drainage already covered. This chapter therefore endeavours to pick up those parts of 'design' not already effectively dealt with, and also to reiterate some factors that are considered worthy of repetition.

The 'design' of a drainage system for an estate is a scheme envisaged by the 'designer' and set down on paper. It is not a theoretical exercise, but one that must be capable of being interpreted, installed and constructed by a builder reasonably conversant with drainage systems.

Above all, it must work to the satisfaction of the client for an indefinite period of time without causing trouble; and it must be relatively cheap to install and maintain.

The 'design' should be made up of a package of information forming the 'contract documents' and should include a design plan, detail sheets and specification; it is not considered necessary to provide isometric drawings.

The designer must remember that he is providing information for the installer to interpret into an actual working scheme; consequently as much information as is possible must be provided on the design plan. The detail sheets provide back up information explaining – in detail – the more complicated parts of the system.

Information must not be vague, in the hope that the installer will make it work; this can lead to extra costs and aggravation between the parties concerned.

The specification must set out clearly and unequivocally the standard of workmanship, the materials to be used, the method of installation and the testing and approval procedures to be carried out before the system will be accepted by the client or his nominated representative.

The project team

To provide a client with a large building complex – such as a hospital – is more

than a single designer can tackle. It is the work of a project team made up of many specialists, such as:
(a) Project leader – usually an architect.
(b) Assistant architects.
(c) Landscape architect.
(d) Interior designer.
(e) Quantity surveyor.
(f) Structural engineer.
(g) Mechanical engineer.
(h) Electrical engineer.
(i) Public health engineer.

Historically architects are trained and responsible for the design of the drainage and sanitation for a building, but often this responsibility, particularly on large projects, is passed to a public health engineering consultant.

It is the duty of all the members of the team to liaise with and assist each other in providing the client with the best possible total scheme at the most economical price.

Public health engineering consultant

It is the responsibility of this consultant to produce a workable scheme; co-ordinated with the other services, the structure and building plan, he must work closely with the other disciplines and submit and explain his ideas to the project architect.

The project architect

The project architect can be likened to the chairman of the board of a large company; it is part of his duty to co-ordinate the work and the final schemes of all the various disciplines to produce a total workable scheme within the cost limits allowed.

The landscape architect

The landscape architect must agree the positions of manholes, the provision of land drains, the possible use of surface water and ponds to create ornamental lakes, which are also useful as static tanks for fire fighting purposes.

If the ground is to be either cut into or filled there will be considerable implications with regard to the way ground water must be diverted.

There may also be implications relating to the invert levels of drains and the authority sewer outfalls, and any pumping that may therefore be necessary.

The quantity surveyor

The quantity surveyor is the cost controller of the project and has to be able to put together a bill of quantities for tender purposes. He will need to know why the system costs what it does, and will be able to 'cost' alternative schemes to discover the cheapest.

The structural engineer

The structural engineer will be required to provide information on foundations, columns, beams, floor construction, ducts and lift wells.

The drainage pipework must be capable of leaving the building and may therefore require passage through the structure.

The floor will require penetrating with wastes and stacks, and any beams must have access through them to allow for horizontal drain runs.

Vertical ducts often come down the height of a building alongside columns, but it is considered preferable to come down away from the structure as column bases can be extremely difficult to negotiate if their top surface is not at least 1.5 m below ground level.

A method of fixing the pipework systems from the structure must be agreed with the structural engineer, and possibly co-ordinated with the requirements of the other services engineers.

Dependent upon the depth – if any – of the inter-floor ceiling zone, vertical ducts will be required for drainage at places selected by the public health engineer in consultation with the architect.

Greenwich district hospital (Fig. 8.1) had between each floor a 2.13 m structural zone, leaving a 1.7 m service void between the upper and lower reinforced concrete slabs. As well as containing engineering services, including drainage, air conditioning ductwork and other services, it provided access for maintenance to all the services.

Although this was an 800-bed hospital there were only three vertical shafts gathering together the horizontal services and allowing access to vertical drainage stacks. This type of ductwork may be considered expensive today, but it did provide near ideal conditions for all the engineering services that accounted for nearly 50 per cent of the total building costs.

However vertical ductwork is provided it must not dictate that the drainage is offset at each floor.

The mechanical and electrical engineers

It is essential that those responsible for the design of these engineering disciplines collaborate and co-ordinate with the public health engineer.

Drainage is the only service relying upon gravity for transportation; all the others use pressurized systems. Drainage therefore requires a gradient, and because of this can cause co-ordination problems. Air conditioning ductwork also has space problems related to the size of the ductwork and cannot easily be moved to accommodate the drainage. Co-ordination is therefore the essence of

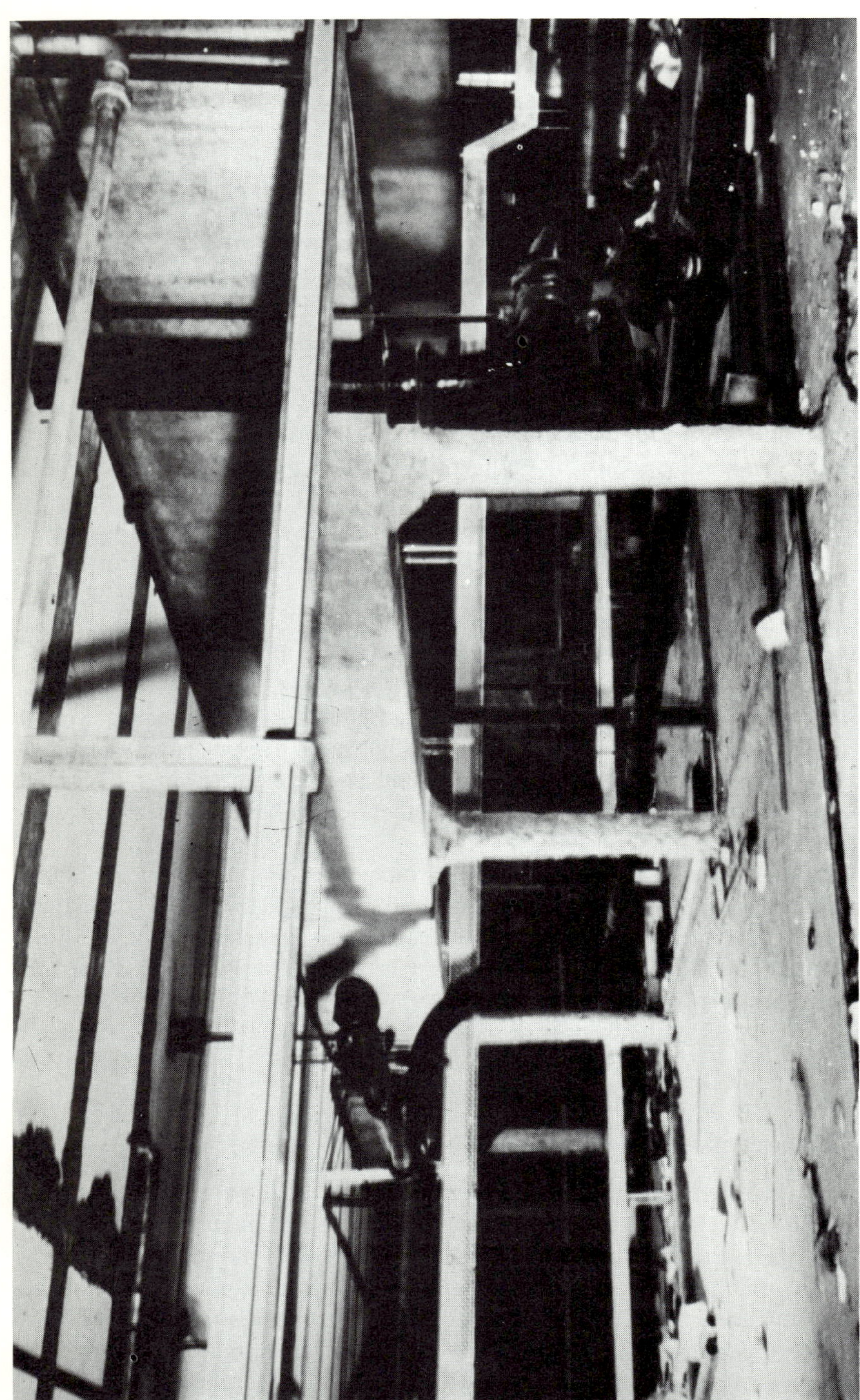

Fig. 8.1 Inter-floor/ceiling walkway duct

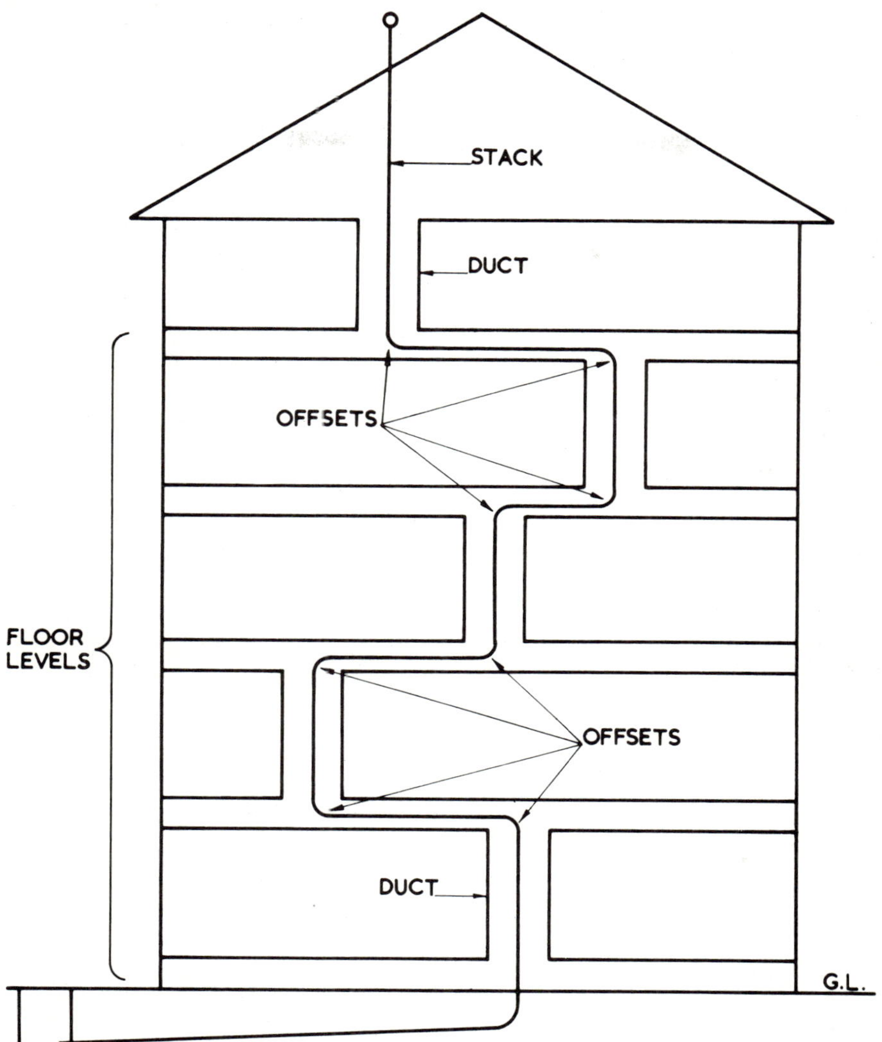

Fig. 8.2 Unacceptable vertical ductwork

engineering services, not only within internal ductwork, but throughout the project.

On large, complex projects it is advisable to produce fully co-ordinated services and structural drawings and details of those areas where the services are particularly complex or congested.

Design process

To provide a workable scheme the designer must be in possession of the site layout, the building plans at all floor levels, including the roof, the structural drawings and sanitary appliance specifications.

The site

Much of the drainage for any estate is likely to be installed underground and it is imperative that the designer investigates the site thoroughly and makes himself aware of any circumstance that may affect the installation or working of the drainage systems.

Obviously the condition of the soil is important in terms of excavation – and, consequently, costs.

Rock will require blasting; it may also be necessary to use rock-breaking equipment.

At the other extreme, made-up ground or a boggy site may require reinforced strip foundations on piles.

The ground water table should be investigated, in both summer and winter conditions, as an allowance may be required for de-watering trenches.

The type of soil will also affect the material used for backfilling trenches, and selected backfill may have to be imported on to the site.

Trees, hedges, ditches, streams and ponds can also affect the design of the drainage system.

The natural movement of ground water must be allowed for and any irrigation or land drainage pipes or channels picked up and re-routed.

Building plan

The drainage designer will require plans at about 1 : 50 scale of every floor level of the building with the positions clearly marked of each sanitary appliance or item of equipment requiring a drain outlet or connection.

After studying the plans he must produce outline drawings showing proposed drain runs related to the structure and then discuss with the architect the requirements for vertical and horizontal ducts. He must also consider the provision of roof drainage and any other areas such as balconies that may require surface water connections.

These plans must also be passed to the other engineering designers for coordination purposes. It is unlikely that the first design will be accepted, but it is the beginning of the 'design exercise'.

The type of roof is obviously important – flat, pitched, or multi-pitched, requiring valley gutters.

At this time he must also consider the implications of the fire regulations relating to the penetration of pipework through compartment walls and floors.

Sanitary appliance specification

Often the architect or even the client will choose the sanitary ware, sometimes on the basis of colour and shape rather than functional use or efficiency. It is, however, important that items of equipment and sanitary appliances are selected early in the design stage so that their outlet positions and dimensions can be checked for compatibility with the structural penetrations and fixings to partitions. During this process the designer must always be aware of the types of effluent the pipework systems will have to carry and consequently the material he is likely to use, which in turn will affect the choice of support system. He

Table 8.1 Maximum fixings for drainage pipework materials

Pipe materials	*Pipe size*	*Vertical spacing*	*Horizontal spacing*
Cast or spun iron	All	3.0	1.8
Copper	25	2.4	1.8
	32/40	3.0	2.4
	50	3.0	2.7
	65/100	3.7	3.0
Galvanized steel	75	4.6	3.7
	100	4.6	4.0
MUPVC	32/40	1.2	0.5
	50	1.2	0.6
Polypropylene	32/40	1.2	Continuous
	50	1.2	0.5
	100	2.0	1.0
upvc	32/40	1.2	0.5
	50	1.2	0.6
	75/100	1.8	1.0
	150	2.0	1.2

must also plan the access points for drain maintenance so that they are accessible through the structure, the other services, and are acceptable to the client. At this time he should consider the production of the Planned Maintenance Manual.

Fire precautions

The statutory fire precaution requirements related to the penetration of drainage pipework through compartment walls and floors are laid down in Section E12 of the Building Regulations and must be followed.

There is, however, much emotive discussion and uninformed opinion regarding the use of 'plastics' material, little of which is based upon test data.

In terms of fire risk the materials used for above-ground drainage purposes can be divided roughly into three categories.

(a) All metals – except lead, and including glass.
(b) PVC compositions.
(c) All other plastics: polypropylene, ABS, etc.

The first category of materials presents no real fire-related problems as they are not flammable, create little toxic fumes and do not fall away from their fixing systems.

PVC type materials are not comparable with the other plastics materials as they are difficult to ignite at normal fire temperatures and readily go out when the flame source is removed. With very hot fires and in the presence of oxygen PVC will easily burn and hydrogen chloride and carbon monoxide are produced; these gases are toxic and irritating to the eyes and respiratory organs.

When correctly supported with metal fixings fire tests show that PVC tends to intumesce, forming a hard brittle coating, often closing the diameter of the pipe to the passage of fumes.

Polypropylene and ABS easily burn in the presence of fire and they can drip burning particles, progressing the spread of the fire. They add to the fire load of a building.

Ad hoc fire tests have shown that GRP bonded to a PVC pipe passing through a compartment structure can form a more effective sleeve than many other materials. The sleeve should be at least 0.5 m either side of the structure.

Stacks fitted with Durgo air admittance valves did not act in the same manner as open stacks; the valve effectively prevented the collapse of the stack for longer than the period of time required by the regulations.

This was also the case of waste penetrations when fitted with a water-filled trap or a rodding point; and, a point not covered by the regulations, a shrouded 'S' trap WC effectively covered the floor penetration and did not fail under the test conditions.

Pumping

The pumping of surface water or sewage will be necessary when

(a) the lowest point in the estate drainage system is below that of the authority sewer or the surface water outfall – stream or sewer.
(b) a collection sump has to be provided to deal with any spillage that may occur below the main drainage system.

These conditions can occur when a building or estate is in a valley below the level of the main sewer system or has a basement below sewer level. It can also occur when the design has a length of drain at such a gradient that the outfall cannot be kept above sewer level. If this occurs during the design stage an attempt must be made to raise the outfall level by either redesigning the networks or changing the gradients.

It must be emphasized that pumping is not only expensive in terms of equipment and accommodation but is also a continuing cost on the running and

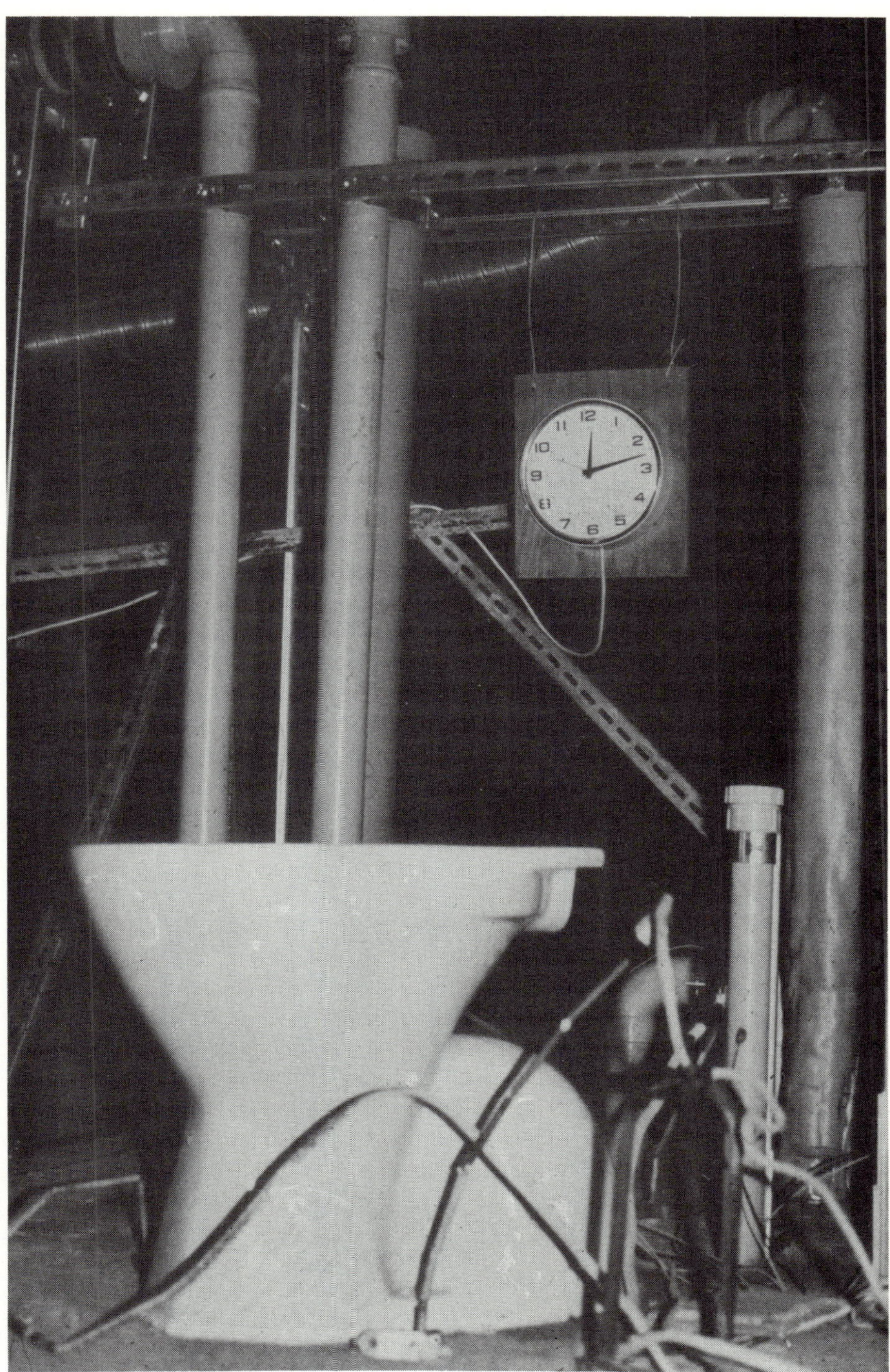

Fig. 8.3 Shrouded WC and Durgo valve on fire test rig

maintenance of the station.

It is recommended that for all pumping requirements two pumps are specified and their use should be alternated with the added facility of one pump being the standby unit in case of the failure of the other.

Pumping methods

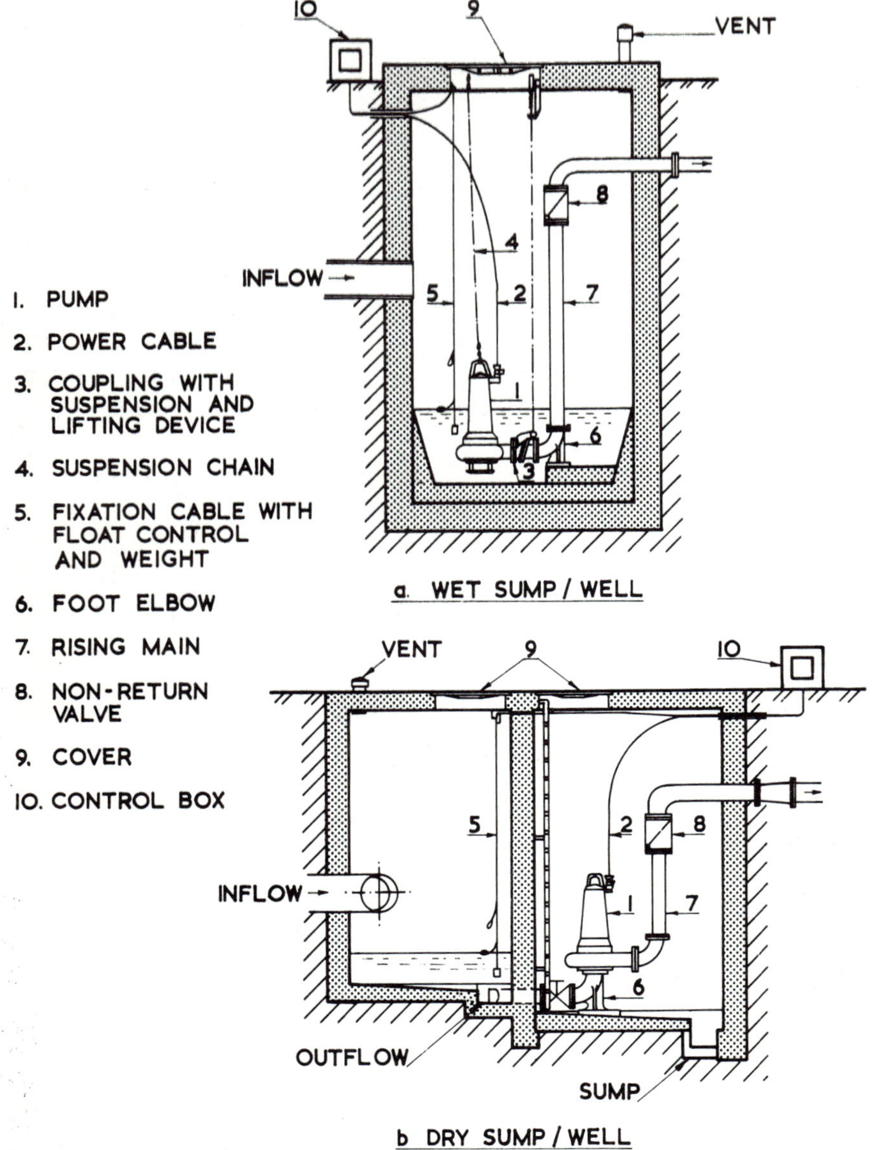

Fig. 8.4 Examples of wet and dry sump wells

There are two basic types of effluent pumping:

(a) Wet well/sump.
(b) Dry well/sump.

The wet well system is where the pump is actually submersed in the effluent. The pump is contained in a sump into which it is lowered and raised for cleaning and maintenance. Some provision must be made for coupling it into the outfall rising main. It is advised that this system is only used for small flows from isolated appliances; it is more suitable for the removal of surface water, or spillage from equipment. Its main economic advantage is that it only needs one chamber. The dry well system is where the pumping equipment is contained in a separate chamber from the effluent. It is obviously more expensive in terms of excavation and structural construction, but is to be preferred from the maintenance aspects of the installation as the pumps and associated equipment can be worked on without disrupting the pumping operation.

A refinement of the dry well system using one structural chamber is the package diverter which is a self-contained unit capable of dealing successfully with small flows of unscreened sewage from communities of up to 1000 persons. One major advantage of these units is that only a chamber has to be provided by the main building contractor, the remainder of the pumping installation being supplied and installed by the specialist company nominated for the work.

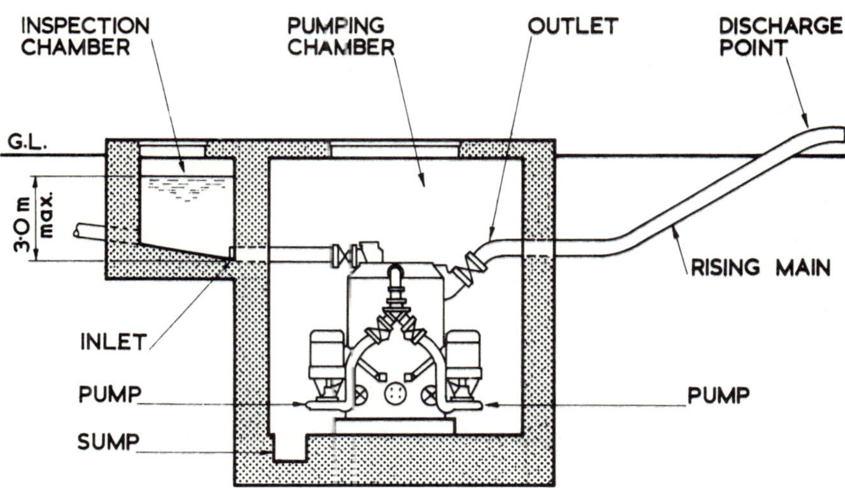

Fig. 8.5 Diverter pumping system

Package pumping stations

Main pumping stations can be constructed either above or below ground, but as part of the system the tanks have to be below ground anyway, so there is considerable environmental merit in placing the whole of the system below ground.

Package pumping stations have been used since the early 1920s, using cylindrical cast iron sections for the outer casings. The introduction of corrosion-resistant coatings allows the use of mild steel as the main structural material and has led to the development of the present-day units – complete pumping stations, factory built with all mechanical and electrical equipment installed, fully tested, delivered to site ready for insertion into the prepared hole and connection to the main drains.

Such chambers can be installed in waterlogged or made-up ground, but there is normally a small amount of civil or structural engineering required dependent upon the size of the unit and the ground conditions.

One manufacturer who specializes in these units constructs two basic sizes 2.45 m and 3.05 m in diameter to meet various pumping requirements at flow rates up to 150 *l*/sec. Two pumping sets are incorporated on a 100 per cent mutual automatic standby basis.

Excavation and back filling

The measure of the success of an underground drainage installation can be judged by the number of times the system blocks, and this can be directly related to the material chosen and the quality of the excavation installation and back filling of the trenches.

It is therefore of prime importance that the trenchwork is to a good standard if later troubles are to be avoided, as any drain failure is disruptive. When it happens below ground it can be very expensive to rectify, particularly if it is under the building, a road or paved area.

The various types of drainage materials discussed are either flexible over their total length such as unplasticized PVC, or rigid and only flexible at the jointing system, i.e. clayware, glass and spun iron.

Flexible pipes

If unplasticized PVC is not correctly installed it can become oval in time depending upon the quality of the installation, the vertical load, the firmness of the surrounding fill and, to a smaller extend, the stiffness of the pipe walls – which can be affected by the temperature of the effluent being transported.

Because the spoil excavated from the trench may vary in its consistency it is usually difficult to successfully compact it around the walls of the pipe and therefore only granular fill is recommended for this purpose.

For practical purposes nominal single sized aggregate or graded aggregate to BS 882 should be used for bedding and side fill to the various pipework materials; selected fill should then be used and well compacted before the main back fill is commenced.

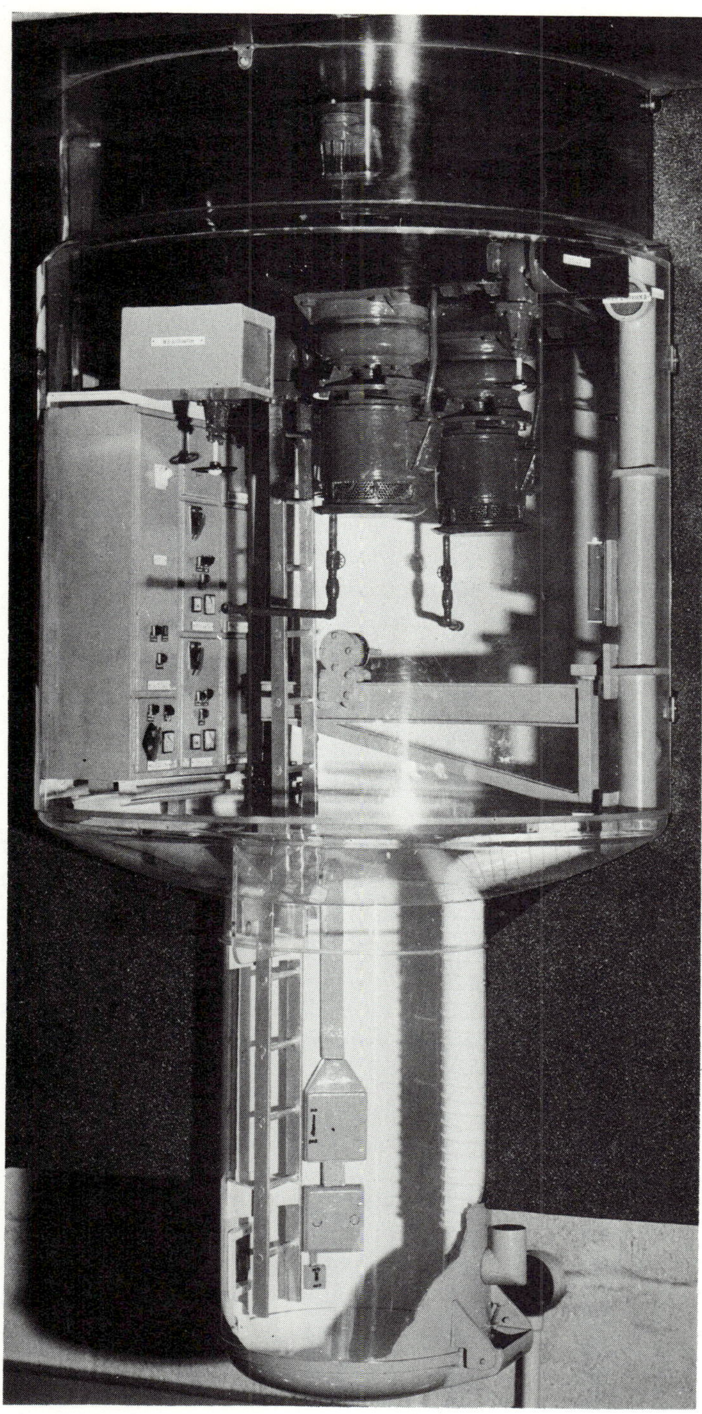

Fig. 8.6 Model view of Package Pumping Station

Table 8.2 Aggregates sizes for bedding and fill

Nominal single size	
100 mm pipe	10 mm aggregate
150 mm pipe	10 mm or 14 mm
225 – 300 mm pipe	10 mm, 14 mm or 20 mm
Graded aggregate	
150 mm pipe	14 to 5 mm graded
225–300 mm pipe	14 to 5 mm or 20 to 5 mm graded

Note: The maximum size should not be exceeded.

Rigid pipes

Most rigid pipes now have flexible jointing systems of some type, allowing movement at the joint and rapid assembly in all weather conditions.

It is particularly important with rigid systems that when a pipe passes through a structure, including a manhole chamber, that a flexible joint is placed as close to and on either side of the structure as is possible; a short length of pipe not exceeding 600 mm should then be used to form a hinged joint allowing for differential movement, as all structures settle slightly.

When a pipe passes through an edge beam or wall it should be sleeved with a clear space around the pipe of about 20 mm which must be cleaned out and sealed at the outer faces with mastic to ensure the space is kept free from dirt and small stones.

There is some risk with long lengths of rigid pipes that differential settlement of the bedding may occur along the length of the pipe allowing it to act as a beam and possibly fracturing due to the vertical load. This should not happen with glass drains as they are encased in a soft plastic outer casing which should take up the deformation, or with spun iron which is 'flexible' to a small degree. If the soil type is suspected of being likely to suffer differential movement, pipes having a length/diameter ratio of 8 or more between joints should be used in lengths within this ratio.

Site traffic

There is a natural tendency to consider that once completed and tested, underground drains can be forgotten as they are protected by the ground above. It must be remembered that heavy site traffic moving over or along drain trenches will compact the back fill and may damage the pipework below, particularly in shallow trenches or those where the surface above is to be made up at some later date.

Defined crossing places must be used and the trench plated over to protect the pipework below.

Combined trenches

The cost of underground drainage is the cost of the completed trench plus a little for the contained pipework. If it is therefore possible to place two pipes in the same trench a substantial saving can be made. It may be difficult, but is not impossible, to design the two systems to have the same inverts, but if the inverts vary a stepped trench can be used.

(a) if the soil is stable enough to stand without breaking down the trench can be cut stepped;
(b) the trench can be cut to the full depth and the difference in level made up with the bedding material.

Stepped drains can be successfully designed and installed, but difficulties may be experienced in the construction of manholes if the difference in the inverts is more than the diameter of the lower pipe.

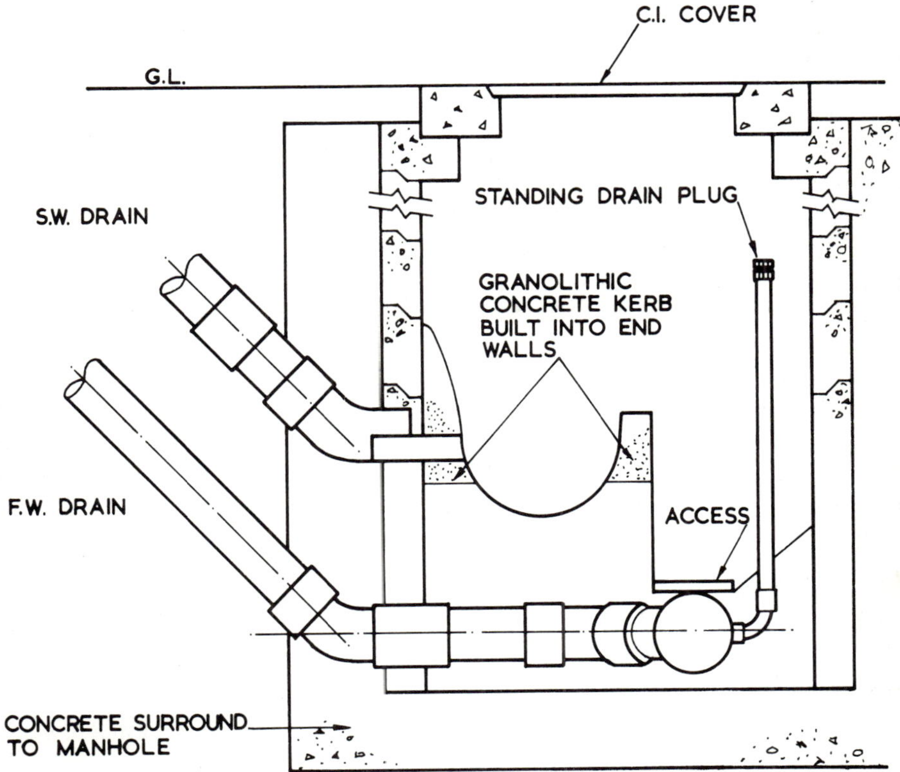

Fig. 8.7 Combined pipe manhole

In Fig. 8.7 the lower foul drain is a sealed system and a standing drain plug is required to drain any surface water that may get into the lower section. The access point could be raised, as in a shallow access chamber assembly to obviate the step in the benching.

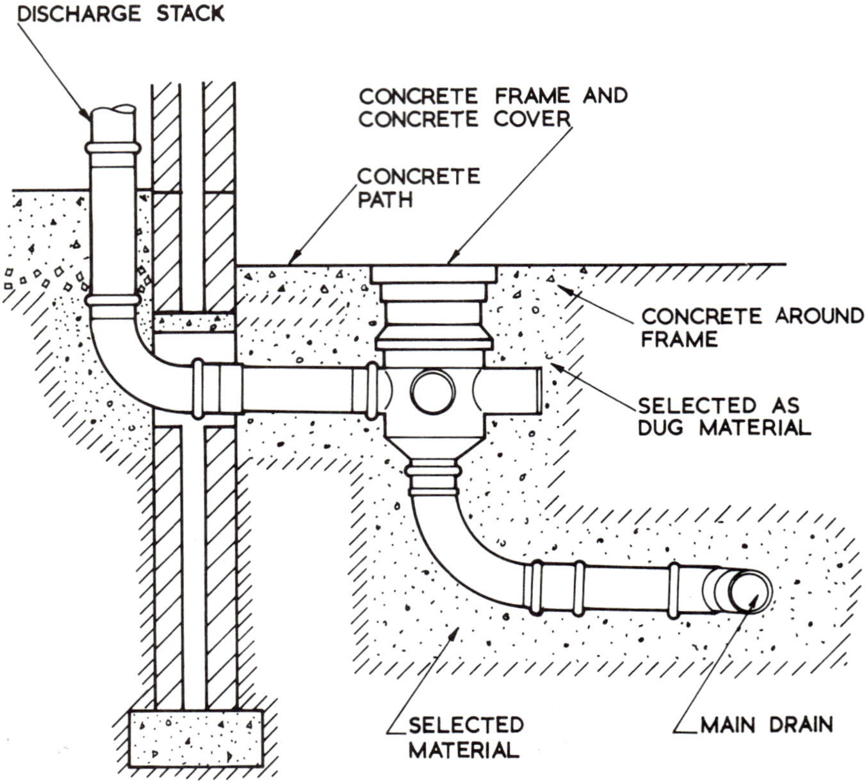

Fig. 8.8 Pipework design: shallow access chambers

Bedding

It is inadvisable to cut a drain trench any wider than is absolutely necessary; the minimum width for any pipe size is the diameter of the pipe plus 300 mm to allow 150 mm on either side for the drain layer to successfully work in the trench.

The trench should be cut at least 100 mm lower than the invert of the pipe to allow for minimum bedding; any over cut can be made up with the bedding, and any soft spots or hollows formed by the removal of large stones or other unacceptable objects must be tamped firm with hardcore.

It is recommended that the bottom of the trench is hand finished to the gradient.

There are other bedding types and methods available, but those shown can be used for most situations and materials.

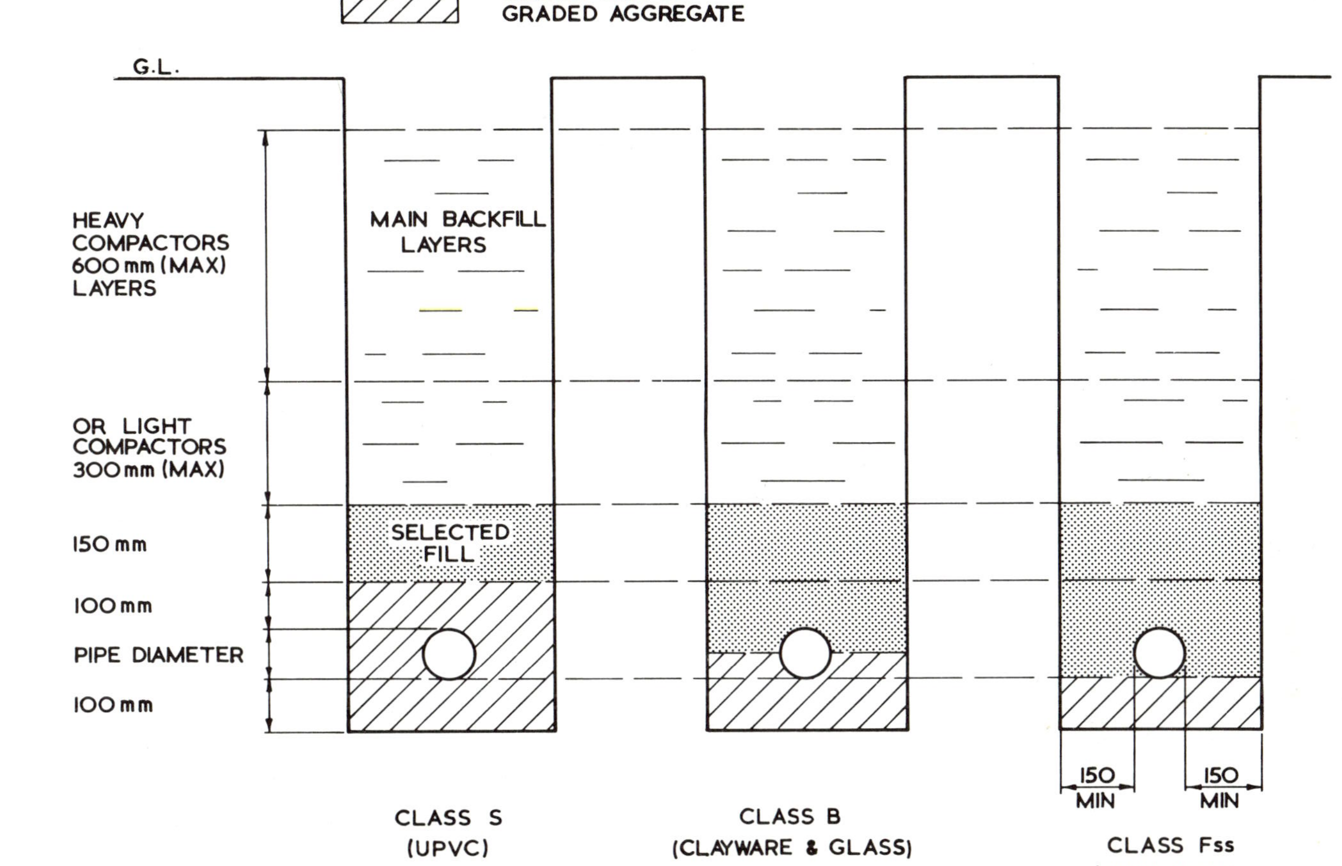

Fig. 8.9 Bedding and backfilling for underground pipework

Class A bedding (not shown). This is a concrete cradle and may be used
(a) where further excavation alongside the drain is likely;
(b) where the pipe is being laid near existing foundations.
By encasing the pipe in concrete a rigid beam may be formed.

Class S bedding is used for unplasticized PVC pipework and where the excavated soil is not suitable for back filling around a pipe because of its formulation. (Surface strip soil should not be used for back filling as it may contain humus which will rot and form pockets around the pipe.)

If the site has a high water table at some season granular bedding can act like a land drain, allowing water to flow along the run of the trench and appear at the ground surface lower down the drain line. To reduce this effect lean mix concrete or puddled clay stops should be provided at the manholes.

Class B bedding is to be used for pipework of rigid wall construction; there is a theoretical saving in using the selected fill from the site, but many contractors prefer to use aggregate for economic reasons.

Class Fss bedding uses less granular fill than the other two methods and is therefore cheaper.

As an alternative to the granular bedding materials specified in BS 882, materials may be used with compaction factors between 0.15 (Class S) or 0.15 and 0.3 (Class B and Fss).

Compaction test

Obtain an open-ended pipe with the ends cut square 250 mm long and 145 to 160 mm internal diameter (150 mm drain pipe is ideal) and a metal rammer 40 mm diameter and 1 kg in weight.

Take a sample of the proposed granular type material by 'quartering' a large sample until about 10 kg is left, i.e. sufficient to fill the cylinder.

Pour the sample slowly into the upended pipe without vibration or tamping until it is completely full and strike off the top level with that of the cylinder.

Empty the cylinder and clean out (it is important that the moisture content of the sample is about the same as the main body of material). Refill the cylinder by placing about one quarter of the sample therein and tamping until it is firm; repeat with the second and successive quarters until the sample has been completely inserted into the cylinder.

Material with a factor over 0.3 is not considered suitable.

Back fill

The drain pipe should be placed on top of the bedding material to the specified gradient so that it is completely supported under the barrel of the pipe for its total length.

The side fill should then be placed in position and lightly hand compacted to ensure that it fits snugly around the walls of the pipe. 150 mm of the selected fill

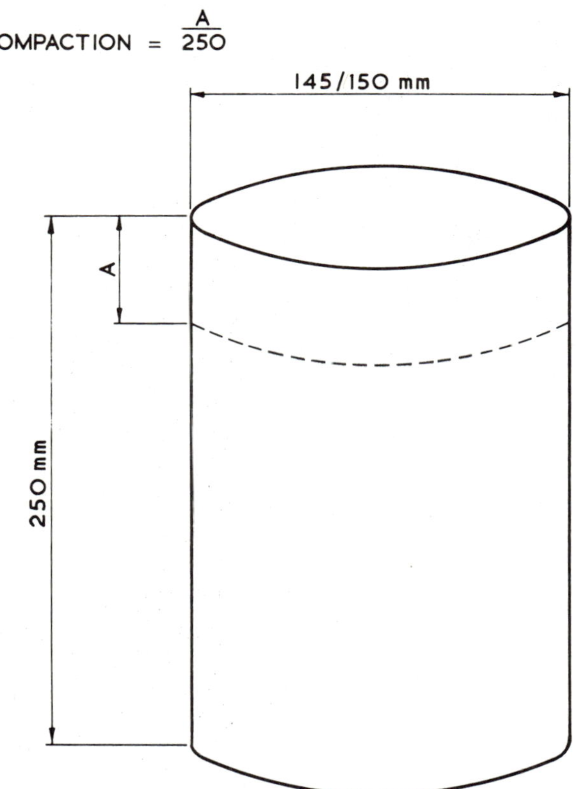

Fig. 8.10 Compaction factor

should then be placed in position and hand compacted, after which the main back fill can be placed in 300 mm layers and hand or light mechanical compaction can be undertaken.

Once there is a minimum of 600 mm of cover over the crown of the pipe heavy compactors can be used on layers of fill 600 mm thick.

The contractor must not tip or bulldoze fill into the trench and any trench sheeting must be withdrawn as the back fill is placed to ensure that no pockets are formed.

At no time should rubbish likely to decompose or tins or drums be used as back fill, or should large rocks, clay or chalk lumps greater than 75 mm be used as fill, as proper consolidation cannot be satisfactorily carried out with these materials.

No trench should be cut and left open to the weather for more than a few hours as it will either

(a) become waterlogged and the bottom soft and unstable;
(b) dry out so that after completion of the works ground movement will occur.

Mechanical excavation

Trenching for drainage is usually undertaken using a front or rear acting hydraulic digger, but for certain types of work a better and cheaper cut can be made using a continuous tracked chain trencher.

These machines can work on grass sites when surface damage must be kept to a minimum. They can cut narrow trenches up to 300 mm wide and 2.5 m deep. They are ideal for land drainage work and long straight outfalls down the slope of a site.

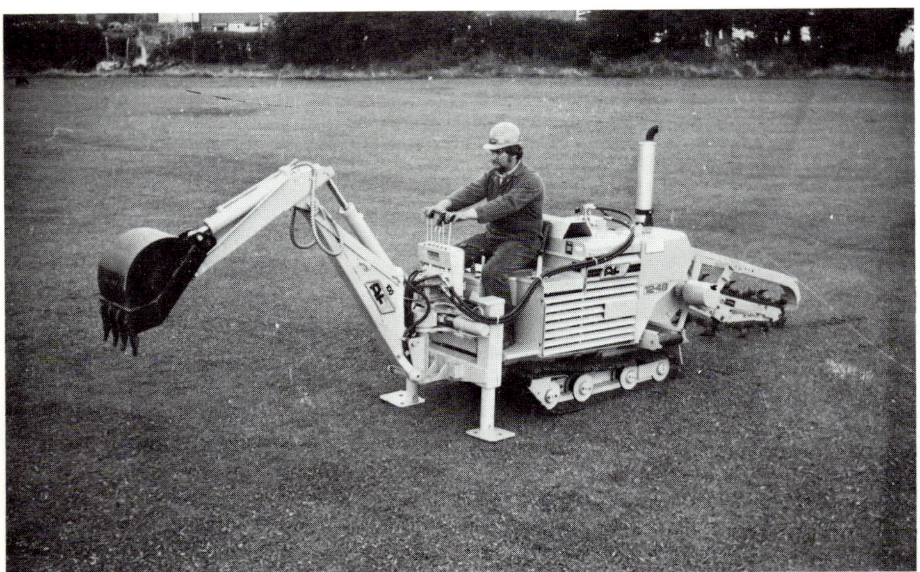

Fig. 8.11 Tracked trencher (back hoe/chain excavator)

Surface water drainage

There are many instances when the designer will wish to control or divert surface water, whether it is in an existing ditch or stream, or just the surface run off from an embankment, sloping field or car park.

The provision of traditional land drainage systems at depths of between 0.3 and 0.75 m is not always appropriate for the prevailing conditions; for example, clay soils will not allow water to percolate into the ground and the water will therefore either lay on the surface or run down the slope to some point where it is held.

During the working of any type of land drain the fine soil particles within the area of the drain will slowly move towards the drain and it is these small particles that slowly block a french drain and sediment up a piped system.

The drainage designer is interested in two basic soil types, granular and cohesive; between these there are a range of mixed soils.

Granular soils such as gravel, sand or crushed rock may have angular or rounded particles and will allow the movement of water through the soil dependent upon the water table, grading and compaction of the particles.

Loosely packed single size aggregates acting as a french drain will allow more water to pass than compacted graded aggregates.

Cohesive soils – clays – can have adjacent negative and positive charges; these attract each other and resist the separation of the particles. These forces give rise to the clay's cohesive strength and thus its ability to resist shear. Clay soils absorb water (tough water), the pores between the particles becoming filled with free interstitial water.

The movement of heavy contractors plant over a site will compact a cohesive soil (but not a granular one), and make it less likely to allow water to drain through the pore structure.

By their nature therefore underground land drainage pipes and rubble-filled trenches slowly sediment up and become blocked. If a rodding point has been positioned at the head of a piped land drain and a mud sump at the bottom the system can be cleaned out, but no amount of maintenance will improved a blocked rubble drain.

Open ditches

Open ditches are often used for lowering the water table or collecting surface water run off from sloping areas.

This method of water collection has two fundamental disadvantages when used in urban areas, the second of which also applies in agricultural areas.

(a) There is a danger of young children falling into a ditch and drowning.
(b) Annual planned maintenance is required to keep the system effective.

With the outward development of estates it is particularly important to realise the danger ditches afford to children and consideration should be given to providing some other means of water collection and removal. There may be a reluctance to spend money on something that is already working reasonably well, but the maintenance cost implications of ditches is considerable.

Small streams and large ditches can be culverted, but the designer must realize that the existing system also allows ground water filtration to occur and it may be advisable to provide along both sides of the culvert a land drain discharging into the culvert via a mud sump.

Filtration fabrics

It has been found from research and site testing that by wrapping the land drainage system in filtration fabric the movement of fine soil particles is effectively prevented from clogging the granular medium and the pipework. The soil next to the filtration medium becomes more permeable due to the movement of

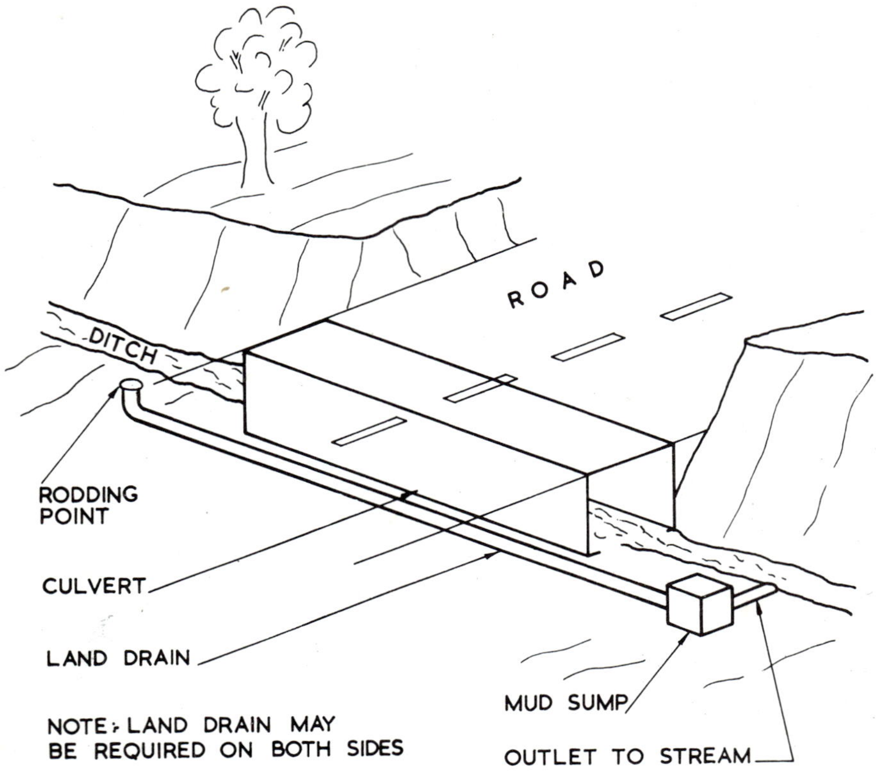

Fig. 8.12 Culvert with land drain and mud sump

particles towards the drain, leaving a more open soil structure, and the migrating particles enter and adhere to the filter fabric, forming bridges through the pores. This process continues until equilibrium is reached when, although the permeability through the fabric will have been reduced, that through the adjacent soil will have been increased.

Filtration fabrics protect the drainage medium and associated pipework system from becoming clogged with fine soil particles over a period of time, thereby reducing the planned maintenance requirements of the system, as well as keeping it at maximum efficiency.

By using it as shown the medium can be covered, eliminating the hazard to pedestrians and vehicles associated with loose gravel. Grass cutting equipment will also not suffer from damage by hidden stones, as children will not be able to scatter them about during play, and the area will be visibly more acceptable than one criss-crossed by gravel strips.

The Althon system

This system of surface water drainage is formed by a semi-trapezoidal duct

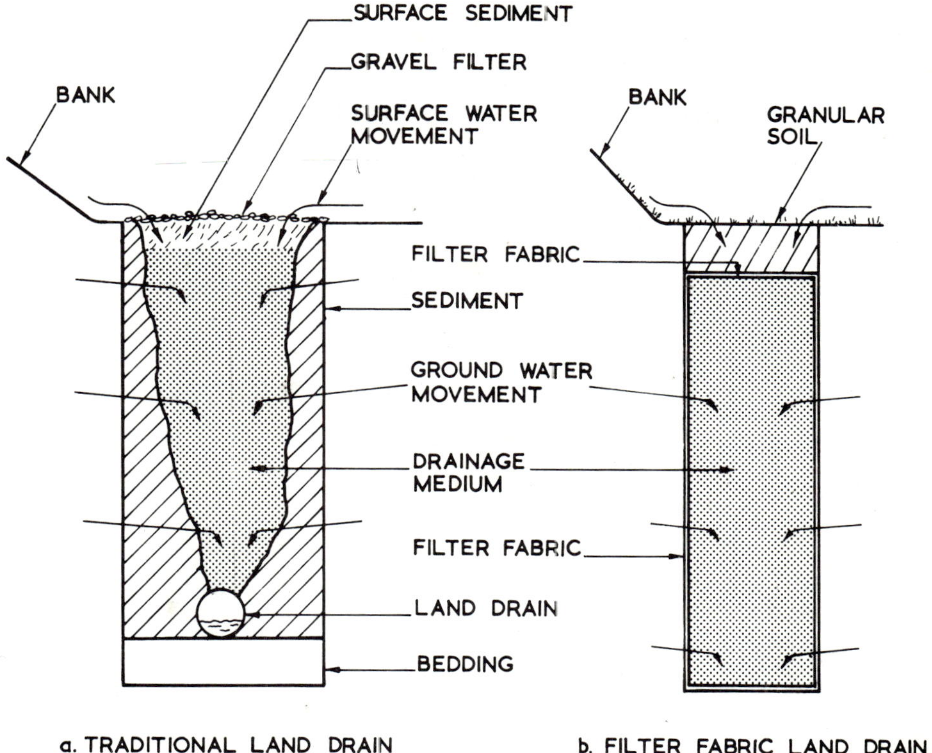

Fig. 8.13 Use of filtration fabrics

which can be used with a kerb or cover, the base of which can be either solid or perforated to allow ground water filtration.

Because the system is installed at ground level there is little excavation and the channel can be laid without a gradient (although one is preferred), and will still maintain a degree of self-cleansing and provide an effective water way and collecting ditch for storm water.

Silt pits should be provided, particularly with the perforated sections before a junction with a sewer pipe.

When used with reclaimed land, artificial or natural embankments it will assist in stabilizing the base of the embankment and also take care of water in the seepage zone.

No fences or other protection is required against animals or children, consequently cultivation or grazing can take place right up to the system.

Above-ground systems

The type of pipework system, either vertical or horizontal, to be used within

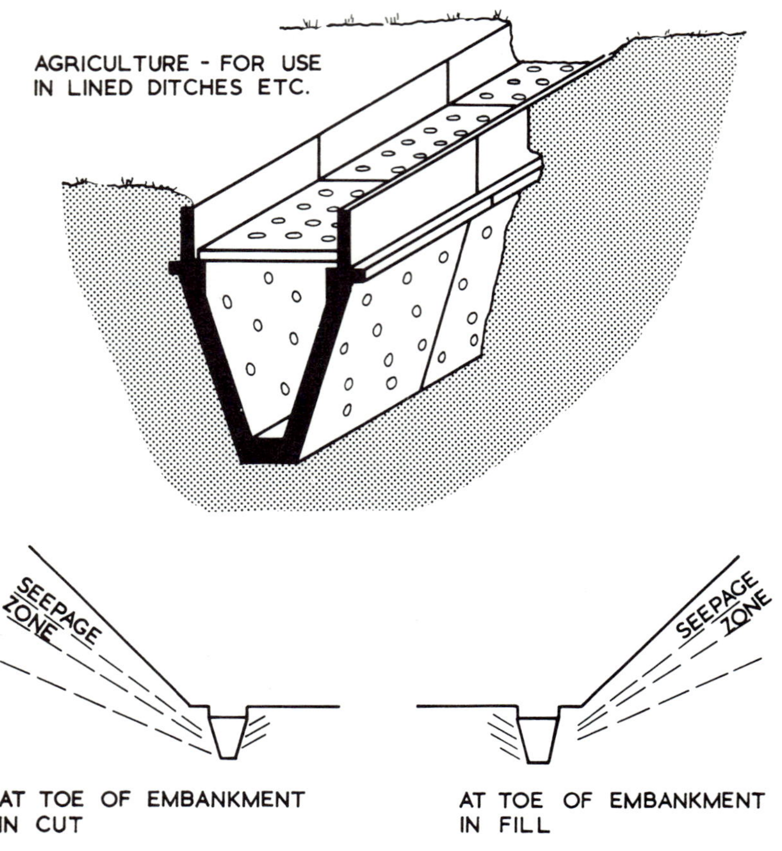

Fig. 8.14 Althon agricultural system

any building type will depend upon the space available for and within service ducts, and the spacing of such ducts over the building plan.

Multi-floor domestic buildings such as flats or hotels, and also offices, should have such ducts sited behind the sanitary accommodation throughout the height of the building. This can usually be designed into the floor plan by grouping and stacking vertically the toilet and kitchen areas.

Depending upon the height of the building and the number of appliances per floor, a simple single stack system of vertical drainage can be applied.

Buildings with large floor plans and open areas such as hospitals should not have the floor planning restricted by numerous vertical ducts required by the single stack system, but should have the scattered sanitary ware linked together by a horizontal system of pipework contained in an inter-floor/ceiling zone.

If possible the designer should attempt to convince the project team that grouping of sanitary accommodation is advantageous, and he should be supported by the quantity surveyor, who will see the cost advantages in such a

Althon units flowing full (to underside of cover)
Extra flow capacity available dependent on height of upstand

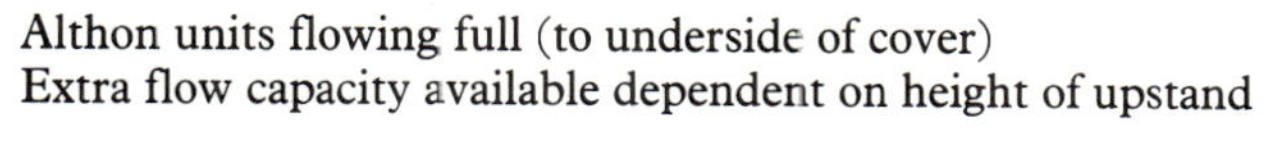

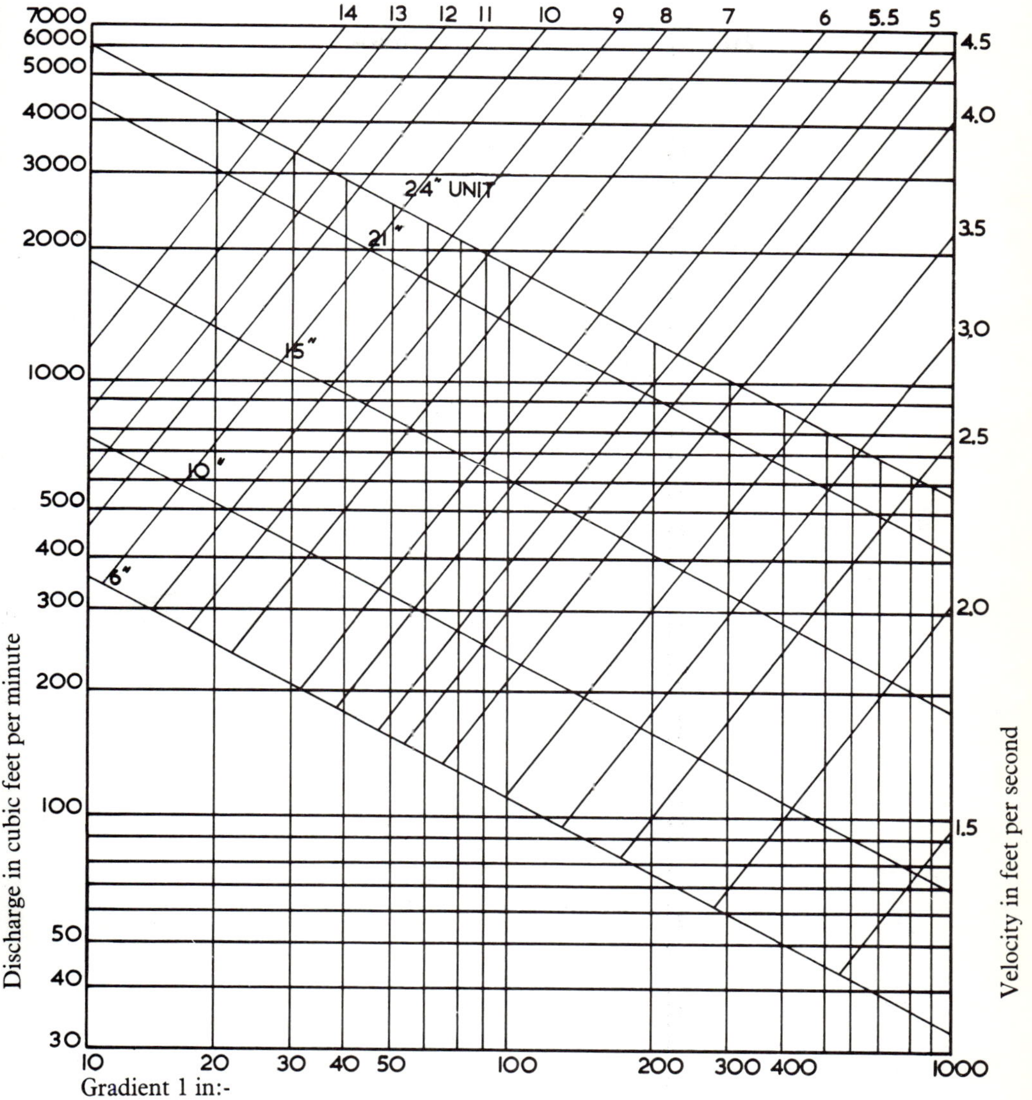

To read: Take point of contact between diagonal line (Althon Unit) and vertical gradient line. Take horizontal line to scale of discharges on left and diagonal line to velocity scale on right.

Based on the 'Manning Formula' adopting an n factor 0.016. This gives $V = 93\ m^{2/3}\ l^{1/2}$ where V = velocity m = hydraulic mean depth and l = hydraulic gradient

Table 8.3 Althon design chart

scheme; but he must not attempt to impose a rigid drainage solution to satisfy his technology to the detriment of the building users' requirements.

Methodology

It is essential that during the planning stage the designer does not forget in his desire to produce a system that fits the building and is acceptable to the project team and the client the basic rules relating to blockages, etc. Duct space is always insufficient, but he should not attempt to squeeze in his system by specifying knuckle bends and offsets: the gradient is not so important if the material and fittings chosen are correct.

The choice of a good fixing system is, however, very important because upon this relies the continuous uniform gradient of the pipework. A poorly designed support system may allow the pipework to snake between fixings and can detrimentally influence the differential thermal movement of the pipework.

It must be remembered that the installation may be undertaken in the below freezing temperatures of winter, but the duct temperature when the building is operational may be in excess of 30 °C.

Access

The designer must discuss and plan with the other members of the project team the type and position of the access points, both into the pipework for maintenance and testing, but possibly more importantly the provision of access through the building fabric to the pipework access points.

Greenwich hospital had an ideal provision for building access but this is not always possible to achieve – particularly with vertical systems.

Access through removable panels or doors must be easy and quick; a full room height 'removable' panel with fifty screws does not meet the required criteria, nor does physically moving or emptying a cupboard to reach an access point.

Obviously effluent should not flood into a habitable or clinical area on the opening of pipe access points; the designer must therefore ensure that they are sited above the flood level of the adjacent sanitary appliances on all main drain runs.

Branch to stack connections

Horizontal branches taking the discharge from WCs, etc., will be at least 110 mm diameter and waste branches of 40 or 50 mm.

If the designer requires that opposite branches joint a stack in the same plane there is a risk of effluent crossing from one branch and backing up the opposite branch. This is less likely to occur with opposite 110 mm branches, but experience has shown that it can occur when a WC branch is opposite to a waste branch.

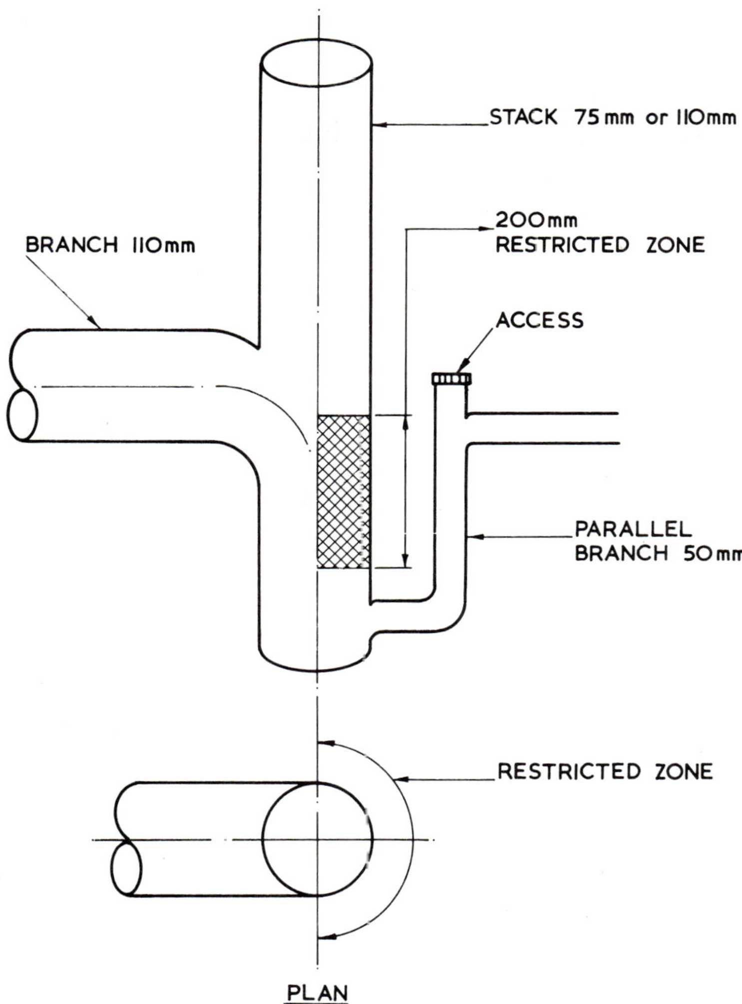

Fig. 8.15 Restrictions on opposite branch connections

There is a restricted zone on a stack where a waste branch should not be connected; if a connection is required, as may be the case with a bath, it should be diverted by the use of a 50 mm parallel branch.

Stub stacks

It has become relatively common practice to use a short 110 mm stub stack to collect the various discharges from appliances on the ground floor of single storey dwellings. This stack must have an access fitting at the top, and from the crown of the WC trap to the invert of the drain must not exceed 1.50 m. and from the topmost connection to the stack and the drain invert more than 2.0 m, or siphonage may occur.

If there are a number of dwellings, all with stub stacks on an 110 mm underground drain, there must be a ventilating stack or traditional soil stack at the head of the run.

Special conditions

Under certain circumstances it is inadvisable to position surface water drainage pipework underground.

Processes that produce a considerable quantity of dirt or dust such as cement works or factories manufacturing precast concrete products can have their underground surface water pipework systems quickly choked with detritus from these processes. This dust will settle on to the roofs of the buildings and on to roadways from where it will be washed into the drainage system by and during rainfall.

The roof gutters will clog, but if they are simple open channels they can be cleaned out by planned maintenance, but down pipes will keep clean if they are offset or horizontal.

The collecting system linking the down pipes should be open channelling crossed by gratings where necessary such as across paved areas or roadways.

The roads should be graded to fall to a method of surface water collection such as the Althon system; gullies should not be used.

Chapter 9

Testing

Objective

The objective of testing a drainage system is to ensure and satisfy the client – and the regulating authorities – that it is sound, watertight, capable of carrying away the effluents that are discharged into it and will function in the installed position for the life of the estate.

The only difference in the test procedure to be adopted for above- and below-ground systems is that the latter must be tested twice, once before and then after backfilling of the trenches. The reason for this double testing is that the first test should show that the system is pressure tight after installation, while the second test shows that the system has not suffered physical damage during the backfilling and compaction of the trenches.

Test procedure

As the testing is usually carried out in stages an 'as installed' design drawing must be marked up showing those sections tested and approved.

The contractor is usually responsible for testing the various systems and each test must be witnessed by the client's representative who should then issue a certificate of approval if the test has been successful.

Any defects shown up by the test procedures must be made good by the contractor at his own expense and to the satisfaction of the client's representative – and that section re-tested. A wise contractor will instigate his own test prior to calling for the representative to witness the official test.

Prefabricated pipework should be tested at the place of fabrication before being shipped to site for installation, where it will again be tested as part of the total drainage system.

Types of tests

(a) Visual inspection.

(b) Air test.
(c) Water test.
(d) Ball test.
(e) Performance tests.

Visual inspection

Every time the client's representative walks over the site he should consciously visually inspect the works being undertaken and must inform the contractor if he sees anything that he does not consider good practice or meets the standard of workmanship laid down in the contract documents.

Drainage underground, once covered, cannot be visually inspected, so the first test, before backfilling, must also be visual as well as physical.

The system must be laid in straight lines and to an even gradient; the pipes must be bedded over their full length on the barrel of the pipe – not on their sockets or spacers. Damaged fittings must not be approved and sockets should, generally, point up stream.

Systems that are fabricated or welded must have expansion joints in the correct positions, and all access doors shown on the design drawings must be correctly placed. It would be extremely difficult to use maintenance equipment through the doors shown in Fig. 9.1 which should have been on the side of the junctions.

At all times the inspector must look for open ends of drains that may allow rubbish to enter the system. If the 'bill' has allowed for approved stoppers they must be used at all times; unsuitable stoppers (Fig. 9.2) must on no account be accepted.

Vertical pipes must be so installed and parallel with the structure, and offsets must not be added to bring together a vertical stack that has just missed its ground slab connection.

The positions of flexible connections before structural penetrations should be checked, as should sleeving, and it is essential to ensure that the gap between a sleeve and the pipe passing through is not filled with grit or stones and properly pointed in mastic.

During construction manholes may become depositories for all sorts of rubbish, some of which may damage the sealed access fittings, and may also enter the system if open channels are used. The contractor may hesitate to fit the cover as he may not have brought the chamber up to the finished level, but he must ensure that some protection is given to the drain and he should be made aware of the fact that he is responsible for cleaning out and making good the systems at his own expense.

Air test

This test is useful for ascertaining the soundness of the joints within the system

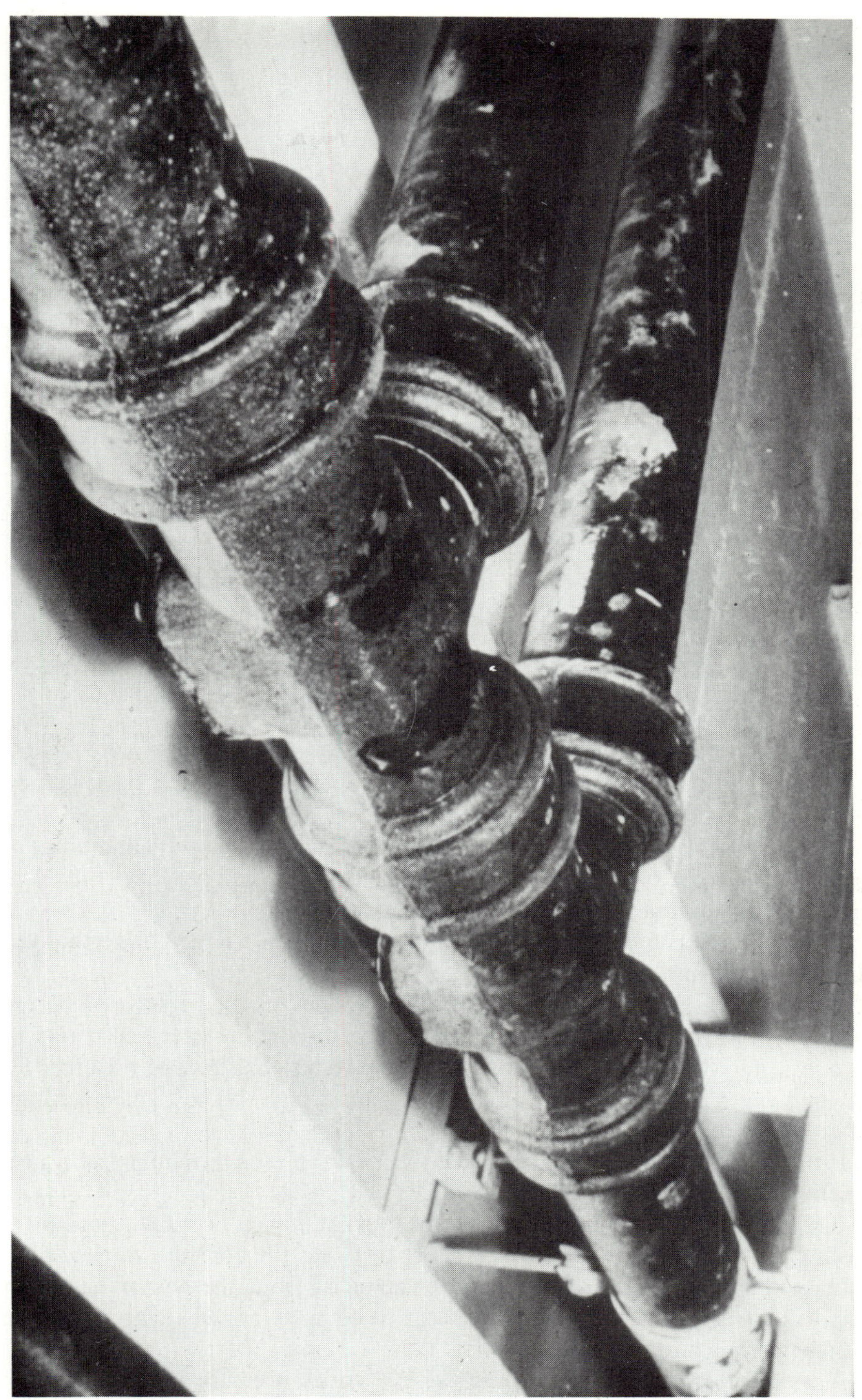

Fig. 9.1 Access door facing soffit

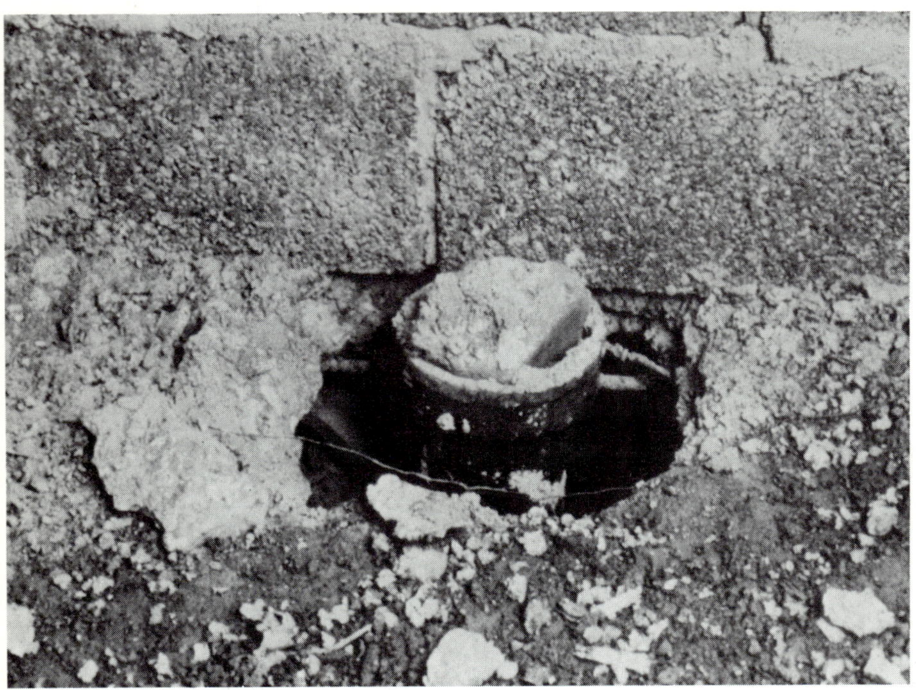

Fig. 9.2 Unacceptable pipe stoppers

and should be completed, if possible, in one operation for each stack or network.

The water seals of each appliance trap must be filled to capacity and plugs or bags inserted at the base of the stack to be tested and at the open end of the vent terminal if an air admittance valve is not fitted.

To ensure the complete seal, a little water may be discharged on to the base plug and the terminal plug greased.

At some point air must be pumped into the system up to a pressure of 38 mm water gauge. This can be achieved by inserting through a water-sealed trap or via a test plug two tubes, one for the air to be pumped through and the other for a manometer connection to measure the pressure, which should remain constant for at least three minutes.

If the air pressure drops it means that there is a leak somewhere in the system which must be found and sealed.

It is sometimes recommended that a soap solution can be painted on to the various joints throughout the system under test with the objective of noting the bubbles that should be blown by the escaping air, but the author has never found this technique effective, particularly in complex systems where much of the pipework is difficult to get at.

A more effective test is to pump smoke under pressure into the system, although this should be avoided with plastic systems. Smoke cartridges must be used with caution and should not be in direct contact with the pipework material as the naphtha used can have a detrimental effect on ABS, unplasticized PVC, and MUPVC and rubber jointing systems. The smoke will be forced out of a defective joint and may be seen or smelt.

Water test

This test is not appreciated by some contractors as they have the problem of obtaining enough water to fill the system and then disposing of the water and possibly mopping up any leakage. It is, however, a preferred test as it simulates what would actually happen in practice if a blockage occurred within the system and it applies a realistic loading test upon the fixing system which is particularly important with horizontal systems.

Pipe fixings must be capable of carrying the dead load of the material and the live load of the effluent, assuming the pipework is full.

Fixings into lightweight concrete soffits must be secure and a test should be applied to a sample fixing by a dead load equal to a 3 m length of cast iron pipe fully charged, i.e. approximately 60 kg for a 110 mm pipe and 110 kg for a 150 mm pipe.

Obviously such a test cannot be applied to a fully vertical system which can only be so tested up to the level of the lowest sanitary appliance, which may be a shower tray or floor gully, when their wastes should be plugged so that the test is applied up to the level of a WC rim.

Test plugs should be inserted into appropriate parts of the system, which should then be filled with water to a level not exceeding 6 m above the lowest plug.

Air will be seen bubbling through the appliance trap seals during this process due to the incoming water trying to compress the contained air.

Underground clayware pipes and fittings may allow some slight passage of air through the material and the absorption of some water; air may also be trapped at the jointing system and some topping up may be necessary before the test water level stabilizes.

If the water level continues to fall after the system has been topped up at 10 min. intervals for 30 min. it must be assumed that there is a leak in the system that will require finding and remedial work.

Manhole chambers should always be water tested to their full capacity as they must not leak out with effluent or in with ground water.

Ball test

To ensure that the bore of the pipework is free from obstruction and that flexible materials have not suffered deformity it is recommended that a ball is passed through the system. A ball 3 per cent smaller in diameter than the pipe should be passed through; if it sticks due to the ovality of the pipework, a ball 5 per cent smaller should be used. If this also sticks progressively smaller balls should be used to establish the degree of deformity of the system.

If the deformity is in excess of 5 per cent the test should be repeated three months after completion of the works to establish the maximum deformation attained, which should not exceed 7 per cent of the pipe bore. If this figure is exceeded a TV camera survey should be carried out to visually inspect the interior of the system prior to deciding what action should be taken.

After this test the whole of the system should be flushed through and performance tests undertaken.

Performance testing

These tests are to prove the design rather than the workmanship as they are a check on the adequacy of the venting provision of the system and the ability of the traps to resist self and induced siphonage.

After each test the traps should be dipped to ensure that a minimum of 25 mm seal has been retained; each test should be repeated three times.

The test should consist of discharging simultaneously a selected number of appliances on one or two consecutive floors and measuring the seal losses on the two floors immediately below those discharging. This type of test really only applies to vertical systems but can be modified to apply to horizontal networks where the appliances discharging must be up-stream of those being tested for seal loss.

Inspection and testing of sanitary appliances

As well as the performance tests for appliance traps there must also be a visual inspection and physical testing of the sanitary appliances.

Visual inspection

This must be carried out after the contractor has removed all the protective wrappings.

Only sound unmarked colour matching appliances or fittings should have been installed and at no time should they have been used to support scaffolding or planking or used for the preparation, mixing, soaking of materials, the cleaning of equipment or tools, or the disposal of waste or unwanted materials.

They should be clean and unmarked by decorative materials and all the fixing screws, bolts or other fastenings must be firmly in position.

The appliances should be fixed level and tight to the wall or partition, with the gap filled uniformly with approved mastic sealant in a smooth uniform manner.

Table 9.1 Performance tests: appliances to be discharged

Type of use	*No. of appliances of each type on the stack*	*No. of appliances to be discharged simultaneously*		
		9 LWC	*Basins*	*Sinks*
Domestic	1 to 9	1	1	1
	10 to 24	1	—	2
	25 to 35	1	2	3
	36 to 50	2	2	3
	51 to 65	2	2	4
Commercial or public	1 to 9	1	1	—
	10 to 18	1	2	—
	19 to 26	2	2	—
	27 to 52	2	3	—
	53 to 78	3	4	—
	79 to 100	3	5	—
Congested	1 to 4	1	1	—
	5 to 9	1	2	—
	10 to 13	2	2	—
	14 to 26	2	3	—
	27 to 39	3	4	—
	40 to 50	3	5	—
	51 to 55	4	5	—
	56 to 70	4	6	—
	71 to 78	4	7	—
	79 to 90	5	7	—
	90 to 100	5	8	—

Floor-standing appliances must be level and square to the wall without packing, and any legs supporting appliances or tops must be upright and properly fixed in position.

Only those fittings and accessories specified should have been installed and their fixings must have been correctly fitted with the appropriate nuts, washers, packings, etc.

Cisterns must be fixed at the height specified and the outlet centred over the flush pipe connections into the appliance.

Hot taps should be on the left when facing the appliance and cold taps on the right and the heads must be correctly colour coded or identifiable.

Wastes should be level and bedded in a waterproof compound with a resilient washer behind the back nut; pop-up wastes should open fully and when closed be watertight. All plugs and chains should be in position.

Physical testing

This should be undertaken at the same time as the final visual inspection and just prior to the handover of the building by the contractor to the client.

All wall-fixed appliances should be tested for the fixing by a small downward pressure on the outside edge of the appliance. There should be no movement at all, for if they do move at that time they will eventually become looser.

Cisterns should have their water level checked by flushing three consecutive times and noting that the switch off fills the cistern to the marked level.

Cisterns should be free from rubbish and the overflows tested by overfilling the cisterns and allowing them to discharge through the overflows.

Plugs should be inserted into all appliances and the taps turned on to bleed air out of the pipework and fill to overflowing the appliance to test the overflow connections. During this test the turn-off capability of the taps can be demonstrated as well as the ability of the plug to hold water.

Shower mechanisms should be tested for the correct pressure and the shower heads or hand showers checked for evenness of spray and that the various junctions do not leak.

All traps should be cleaned out and their seals refilled. During this procedure the nuts should be checked for cross threading.

Discharge tests should be as follows:

(a) Nine-litre cisterns take about 5 seconds to empty.
(b) Baths should be filled to a depth of about 150 mm and should take about 90 sec. to empty
(c) Basins and small sinks should have the plug inserted and the bowl filled to a depth of about 100 mm, the plug removed and the water discharged in about 15 sec.

WCs should be flushed and the wet bowl sprinkled with sawdust. A second flush should ensure that the bowl is totally cleaned and that splashing does not occur.

The pan should not rock on the floor and all fixings should be firmly in position.

Chapter 10

Information: mandatory and otherwise

Introduction

It is the duty of any person involved with the design, construction or installation, maintenance or testing of any form of drainage system to comply with various Acts and Regulations related to drainage and sanitary systems for buildings and estates.
The mandatory rules are laid down in the

(a) Public Health Act 1936, with some additions in the 1961 section.
(b) The Building Regulations 1976, and for those persons operating in Scotland The Building Standards (Scotland) Regulations 1971–1975.

For time to time various additions and alterations are made to these documents and it is advisable to research the latest publications for changes.

Within the 'Regulations' there are 'deemed-to-satisfy' provisions relating to the fitness of materials available for drainage systems, which allows the user of any method of mixing or preparing materials, or of applying, using or fixing materials which conform with a British Standard or British Standard Code of Practice prescribing the quality of material or standard of workmanship to be deemed to comply with the requirements of the 'Regulations'.

It does not in fact cover the 'design' guidance set down in the Standards or Codes, and this is noted in BS 5572 (1978) Code of Practice for Sanitary Pipework (formely CP 304), which states that 'This Code of Practice represents a standard of good practice but compliance with it does not confer immunity from relevant statutory and legal requirements'; and there is some conflict of design information between the Regulations and the British Standards/Code of Practice, primarily because they are not updated at the same time – or by the same committee.

British Standards Institution

The British Standards Institution prepares and publishes under the direction of various committees and under the authority of the Executive Board 'Standards' and 'Codes of Practice' relating to materials and design. Again, from time to time they are updated or revised in relation to technological changes or circumstances; but at all times such changes are in accordance with good practice as judged by the technical members of the committee involved.

The British Standards Institution was formed in 1901 and incorporated by Royal Charter in 1929.

The principal objectives of the Institution as set out in the Charter are to co-ordinate the efforts of producers and users for the improvement, standardization and simplification of engineering and industrial materials; to simplify production and distribution; to eliminate the waste of time and materials involved in the production of an unnecessary variety of patterns and sizes or articles for one and the same purpose; to set up standards of quality and dimensions; and to promote the general adoption of British Standards.

In carrying out its work the Institution endeavours to ensure adequate representation of all viewpoints. Before embarking on any project it must be satisfied that there is a strong body of opinion in favour of proceeding and that there is a recognized need to be met.

The Institution is a non-profit making concern. It is financed by subcription from firms, trade associations, professional institutions and other bodies interested in its work, by a Government grant and by the sale of its publications.

Membership of the Institution is open to British subjects, companies, technical and trade associations and local and public authorities. The Standards/Codes relating to the design of sanitary systems are:

(a) BS 5572 (1978). Code of Practice for Sanitary Pipework (formerly CP 304).
(b) BS Code of Practice CP 301 (1971) (under revision). Building Drainage.
(c) BS Code of Practice CP 308 (1974). Code of Practice for Drainage of Roofs and Paved Areas.
(d) BS Code of Practice CP 312 Part 1 (1973). Code of Practice for Plastics Pipework (Thermoplastics Material). Part 1. General Principles and Choice of Material.
(e) BS Code of Practice CP 302 (1972). Small Sewage Treatment Works.
(f) BS Code of Practice CP 2005 (1968). Sewerage. Originally published as Civil Engineering Code of Practice No. 5.

There are numerous 'Standards' relating to specific materials; and those manufacturers whose materials come within the limits laid down by the relevant 'Standard' can apply to the British Standards Institution for a licence to use the Institution 'Kitemark'.

The presence of this mark on or in relation to a product is an assurance that the goods have been produced under a system of supervision, control and testing operated during manufacture and including periodical inspection of the manufacturers works in accordance with the certification mark scheme of the BSI designed to ensure compliance with a British Standard.

It is important that when selecting a specific manufacturer's product, or allowing the contractor to select materials or components, that only those items

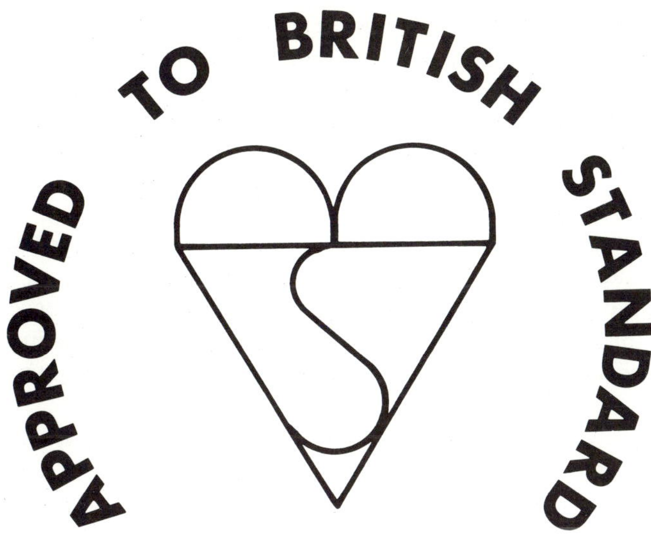

Fig. 10.1 Institute Kite mark

having the BSI Kitemark approval are specified or used, unless they are covered by an Agrément Certificate.

To revise or produce a Code of Practice on drainage may take up to five years as each part must be agreed by the drafting committee whose members are provided by various associations, government departments and institutes and who may have to refer back to other committees who may have a vested interest in any changes proposed.

Many Codes are however based upon the work carried out by the Building Research Station, whose Digests and Current Papers precede new, or changes in, Codes and which provide useful design guidance information.

Agrément Certificates

The Agrément Board is an independent company set up by the Ministry of Public Buildings and Works in 1966.

The Board is principally concerned with the testing, assessment and certification of products for the construction industry in order to secure the ready acceptance of the products concerned and to ensure their safe and effective use.

The subjects for assessment are normally new or innovatory products, but existing products may be assessed sould be need arise; for example, as a result of changes in the building regulation requirements.

The Agrément Board is sponsored by the Department of the Environment (DoE) and its Chairman and Council Members appointed by the Ministry of Housing and Construction.

The following bodies are directly represented on the Board by the appointment of an Assessor:

British Standards Institution.

Building Research Establishment.

Department of the Environment.

Greater London Council.

Scottish Development Department.

The Board receives the fullest possible co-operation from other Government departments and local authorities.

The Board is a member of the European Union of Agrément (UEAtc), whose objective is to facilitate international trade in the building sector; it is interesting to note that many Certificates relate to products manufactured outside the United Kingdom.

A Certificate gives a totally independent opinion of the performance in use of a product, component, material or system.

All relevant performance factors are assessed in relation to a defined-use category, embracing safety, habitability, installation and practicability, durability and maintenance requirements.

Manufacturers of products awarded an Agrément Certificate are subject to quality control surveillance by the Board or its agents during the period of validity of the Certificate.

The Board stands by its opinion of the likely performance of the products certificated and does not seek to exclude liability for negligence in reaching that opinion.

Manufacturers of Agrément certificated products registered with the Board are encouraged to make use of the Agrément symbol. The Certificate relates solely to the product or system defined in that document and may not be related to other products similar in nature, but not covered by the Certificate; they are normally valid for a period of three years, after which time the manufacturer must apply for a reissue of the Certificate which entails reassessment of the product or system in use.

Certificates are not issued for products covered by a British Standard and consequently they form a useful tool to assist a designer in independently assessing the worth of a product or system.

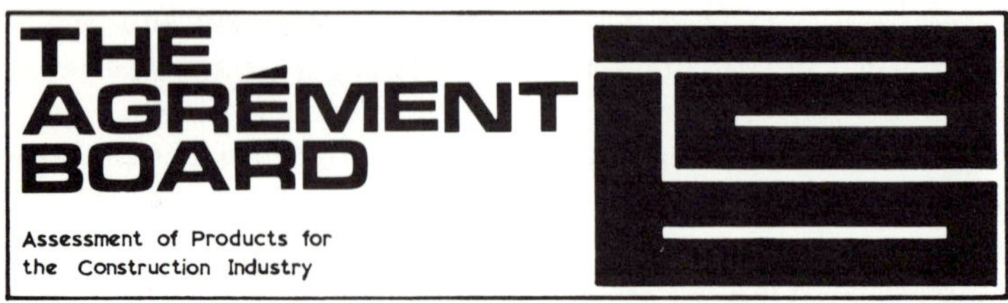

Fig. 10.2 Agrément logo

Building Research Establishment

The Building Research Establishment (BRE) is part of the Department of Environment (DoE) and as such carries out investigations and researches aspects of drainage and sanitation, often culminating ad 'Digests', which in time may become incorporated in Building Regulations or BSI Codes of practice.

It also has an Advisory division which will carry out site investigations into problems related to drainage and sanitation; and in this manner it has built up a vast fund of knowledge which is reflected in its publications. A designer wishing to keep abreast of the latest technical information should ensure that he receives the BRE Digests, and becomes a member of the Agrément subscription scheme for publications.

Trade associations

Trade associations are organizations of individual manufacturers of like products banded together to promote the use and sale of their products.

Many of them carry out research and development on behalf of their members and also provide technical personnel to sit on BSI drafting committees, as well as publish literature related to the use and application of their association's members products.

It must be remembered by designers that these associations are only extensions of individual manufacturer's technical and sales staff, and while they are knowledgeable in the field of their members' products it is the designer who takes responsibility for the selection of materials.

They will usually take up complaints by designers and investigate product failures, as they are also desirous of defending the reputation of their members.

Manufacturers' literature

Most manufacturers of drainage components and systems are conscious that their products must comply with the various statutory regulations and, where possible, to a relevant British Standard, and say so in their literature.

Many manufacturers have expended considerable time and money on obtaining Agrément certificates for their products and systems, including many overseas manufacturers.

They also provide technical design guidance and literature related to the application of their products and systems in terms of Building Regulations and BSI Codes of practice.

Much of this information and advice is excellent, but the designer must not attempt to pass on his responsibility for the scheme he is working on to the manufacturer of the products he intends to use or specify. Although some manufacturers provide a design service, they will not usually take design responsibility, but will accept responsibility only for the replacement of the specific products used.

The cost of replacing a 'failed' product because it has been 'sold' by a manufacturer's agent to the designer is usually only a fraction of the total cost of replacement – and takes no account of the cost of the disruption of the system, or the reputation of the designer.

Chapter 11

Maintenance

General

The maintenance of sanitary pipework systems within a building and its estate is necessary to keep the systems free from blockages within both the pipework and appliances which may prevent the systems functioning as required by the user. The consequences of blockages are disruption to the working of the building, damage to the fabric of the building and a risk to the health of the occupants.

Misuse

Sanitary systems that require maintenance are either defective or being misused.

It is often assumed that a drainage system is like an ever-open dustbin capable of taking any amount or type of waste that is dumped into it and, within limits, this is true. A well-designed and correctly installed system will stand a degree of 'misuse'. Anything that can be discharged through a sanitary appliance should normally travel through the pipework system. If however the system is not in good physical condition, or has been poorly installed or badly designed, blockages requiring maintenance will occur.

Blockages in a drainage system can therefore be attributed to the following, or an interrelation of them:

(a) Misuse.
(b) Design faults.
(c) Poor installation.

Installation

The manner in which a drainage system is installed – as well as the design and use of the systems – can play a crucial part in the degree of trouble likely to be experienced, particularly in the first few months of use.

A good installation specification provided by the designer to the installer is essential. Three clauses that are considered essential in the preambles are:

1. The installer shall at all times prevent the ingress into the system of any object likely to cause a blockage during the life of the system.
2. No object shall be used as a drain stopper except those approved by the client or his representative.
3. The installer shall at his own expense and to the satisfaction of the client or his representative remove and reinstate or clean out any length of pipework found at any time to contain an object likely to cause such a blockage.

The first clause makes it obligatory on the installer to adequately stopper the system. The second informs him that he cannot use plastic bags, etc., as stoppers, and the third lets him know in no uncertain terms what the penalty will be if he is dilatory in these provisions.

Under testing of the systems it should also be a requirement for a ball test to be carried out to ensure that the systems are clean. This test should be undertaken just prior to the hand-over of the building.

Design

Defects in design are either due to a lack of knowledge by the designer or changes in use of the system sometimes caused by alterations or additions to the appliances connected to the system.

A typical example of this is the addition to a ground floor kitchen sink of a waste disposal unit, when the waste pipework is left connected into a back inlet gully which blocks due to the discharge of macerated solids.

Such disposal units should be directly connected into the drainage system, using a standing waste.

Another 'design' defect is the use of manholes with open channels. Evidence suggests that blockages will develop due to items lodging on the benching and falling back into the system. It is also possible that when a manhole cover is lifted, either by an authorized person, or by others, that rubbish may enter the system and create blockages.

Other design defects that are known to cause blockages are right-angle junctions, and knuckle bends that do not allow the free flow of effluent at changes of direction. The inappropriate use of pipework materials can also be classified as design defects.

To create good flow conditions in a sanitary pipework system the effluent must not be impeded by obstructions.

Surveys have shown that in design terms these are:

(a) Right-angle junctions.
(b) Knuckle or acute bends.
(c) Rough bored pipework material.
(d) A jointing system that does not properly align to the pipework.
(e) An ineffective fixing system for above-ground pipework.

CORRECT METHOD

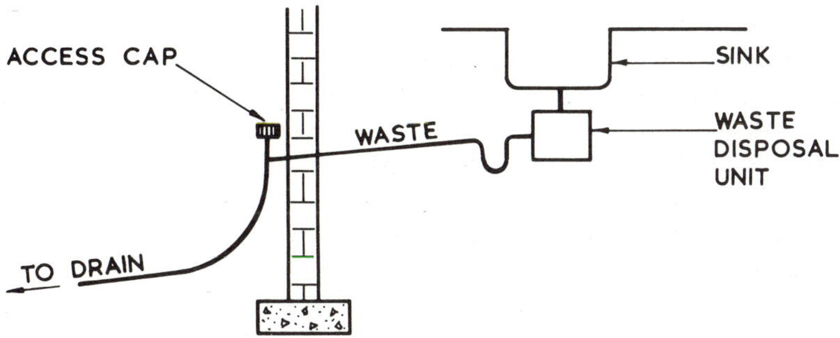

INCORRECT METHOD

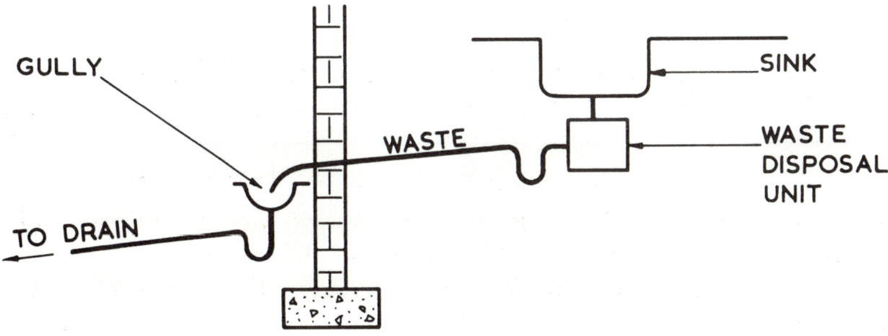

Fig. 11.1 Correct and incorrect method of connecting a waste disposal unit

Rough bore pipe and fittings and a system that does not accurately align the spigot and socket between components will always cause blockage to occur. Solid items, such as paper, etc., will catch on the roughness and create an embryo blockage.

Another type of design defect is the lack of flow from an appliance, coupled with any of items (a)–(e) above. If an appliance does not create good flow conditions within the pipework a build-up of waste can occur and the pipework will slowly block, or, if the amount of waste held in suspension is high, it may not be cleared properly by the water and settle out in the invert of the pipe.

Two examples are:

1. The discharge from a spray tap is about 4 pints per minute (2.27 litres) and runs freely without a plug. Consequently this trickle of water will dissipate and in long wastes will leave the fine solids behind which will build up and slowly block the pipe. This does not mean that spray taps should not be used, but that the design of the waste pipework should take account of the

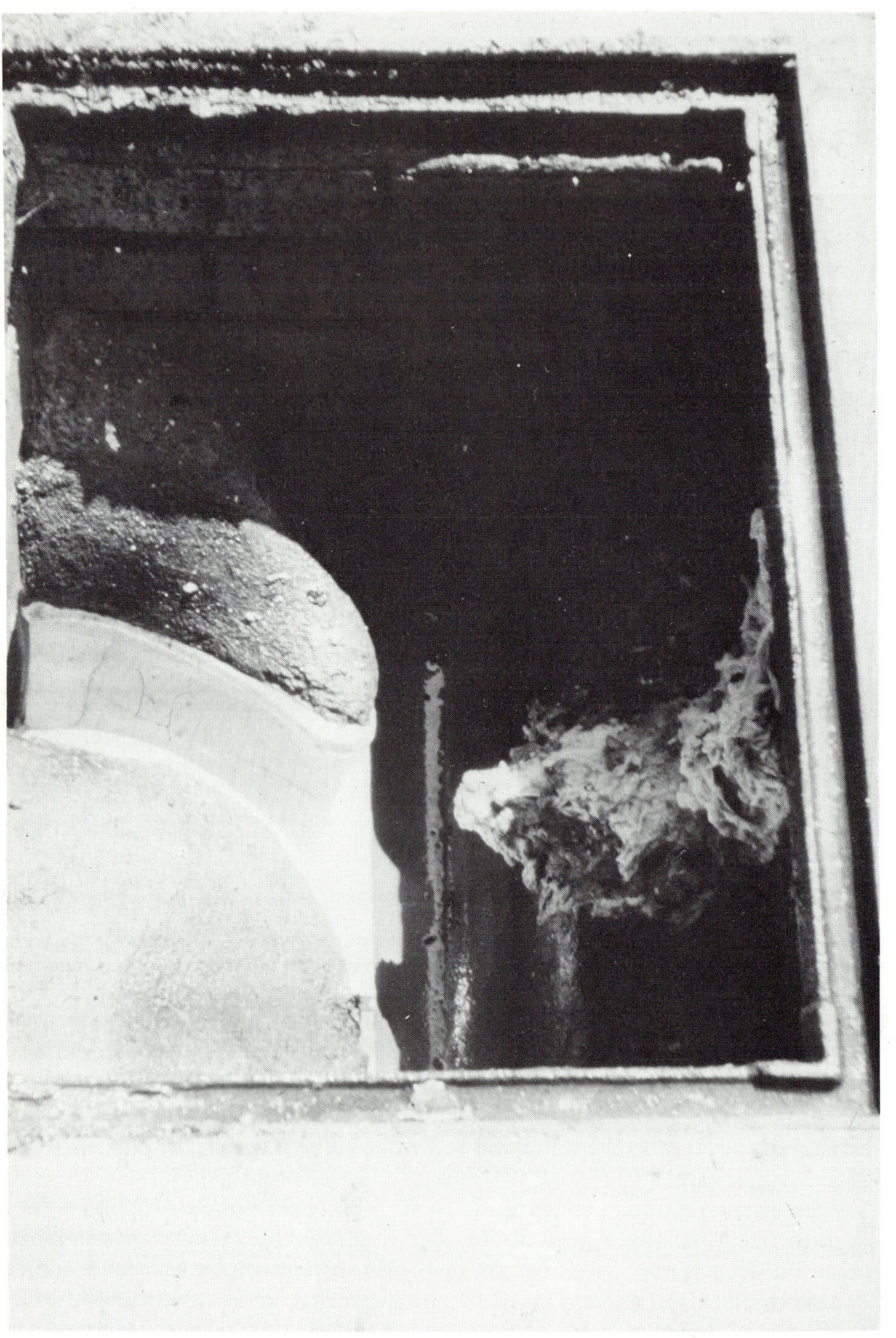

small flow by being short in length, less than 3 m, and of steep gradient (more than 1 : 50).

2. In hospitals, papier-mache bedpans are destructed in a special disposal unit. If this machine is misused or the water supply is inadequate the macerated waste will be discharged like porridge and consequently block the waste system.

A fixing system that does not adequately support the pipework system in an horizontal service void will add to the risk of blockages developing irrespective of the pipework material.

By allowing looping of the pipework, conditions of back flow will occur and effluent will rest and solids settle out within the loops.

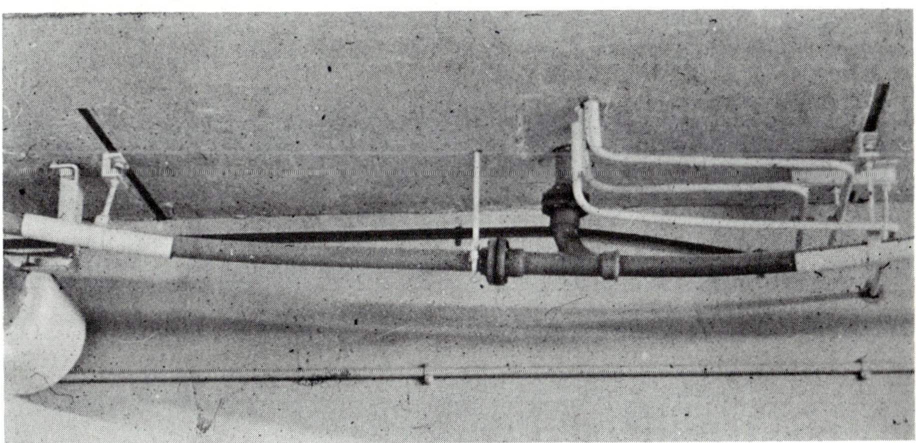

Fig. 11.3 Inadequately supported pipework system

As material plays such an important part in the number of blockages within a system it is important to note that there is a simple performance specification for all sanitary pipework materials to prevent blockages. A well designed and installed fixing system will hold the pipework at the gradient the designer intended to ensure adequate self-cleansing flow.

The pipe and fittings must be as follows:

(a) Of smooth bore.
(b) With well radiused fittings.
(c) Joints that align the spigot-sockets to engineering tolerances.

The most widely used material that currently meets this specification is PVC, both above and below ground.

For chemical effluents it is advocated that the use of borosilicate glass pipework should be considered.

Fig. 11.2 (facing page) Build-up of waste on manhole benching

It has been noted that where these materials have been used blockages due to design have been minimal.

Effects of blockages

A blockage that develops in a sanitary system has two main effects:

1. That if the system is continued to be used effluent will appear within the building at sanitary appliances above the blockage.
2. This effluent and the process of cleaning will release pathogens into the building with the consequent risk to health.

Blockages rarely occur in vertical stacks; they are created in horizontal pipework at changes in direction, junctions and joints between components.

Usually the first indication of a blockage is blow back through an appliance seal due to back pressure. This is followed by the effluent backing up and flooding the appliance and spilling on to the floor.

The first duty of any person suspecting that a blockage has developed is to stop appliances from being used, as their continued use increases the effluent in the system. They must then inform the person responsible for maintaining the system, call in specialist contractors or clear the blockage themselves.

This cleaning operation should be undertaken through access points built into the system specifically for the purpose.

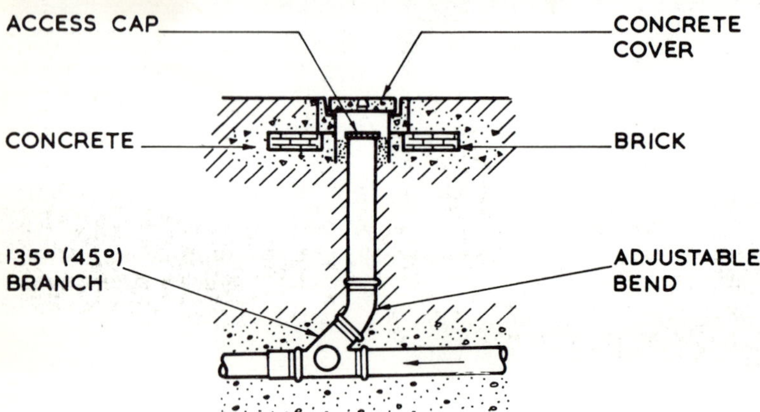

Fig. 11.4 Typical rodding point for maintenance purposes

Effluent can be pathogenic, corrosive or radio-active depending upon the type of equipment attached to the system. It is always disgusting and messy.

The clearing of a blockage is a task that requires some training and, in large estates with complex drainage systems, also a knowledge of the layout of the systems and the positions of the access points.

Two aids in the process of maintenance are:

1. A drain blockage indicator which gives a visual or audible warning of a blockage in a horizontal pipe before it appears at an appliance.
2. A sealed rodding point that allows maintenance to be carried out either below flood level, i.e. in a basement, or in a sensitive area of a building, such as a kitchen, without opening the drainage system.

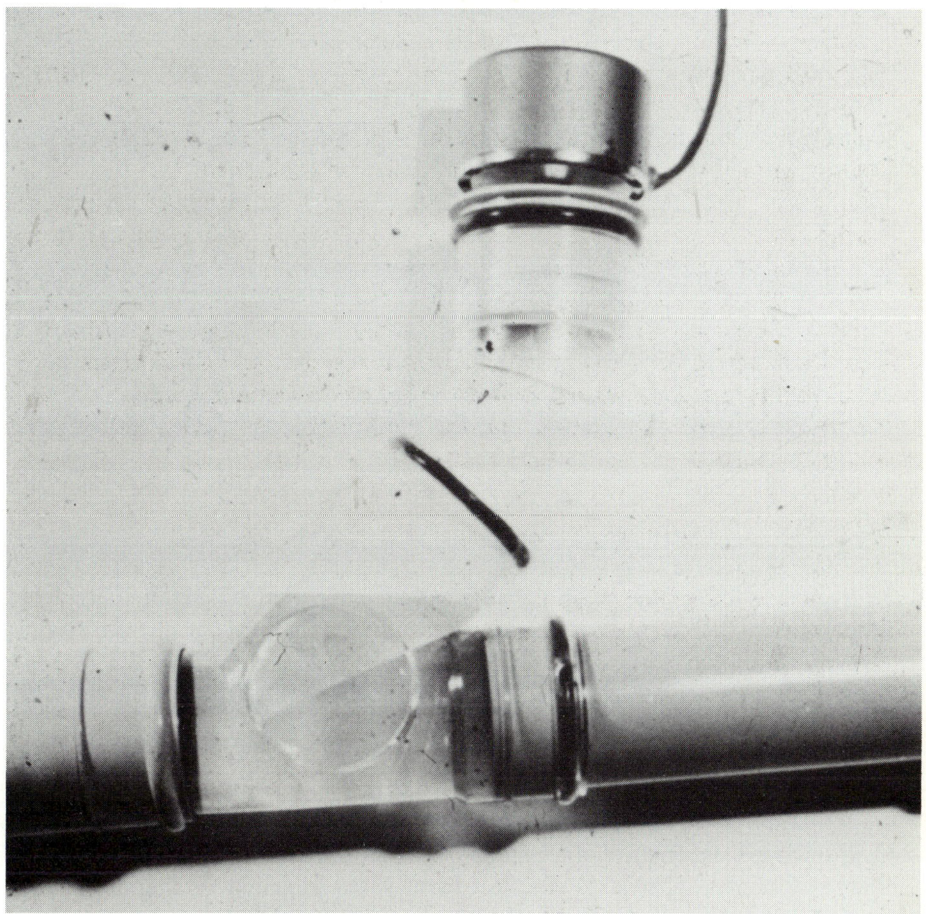

Fig. 11.5 Drain blockage indicator

As effluent is potentially dangerous, maintenance personnel carrying out routine procedures must be aware of the effluent they are likely to be dealing with. They must be trained, provided with the appropriate equipment and protective clothing and regularly medically checked.

Medical advice must be given to drain maintenance staff on matters of per-

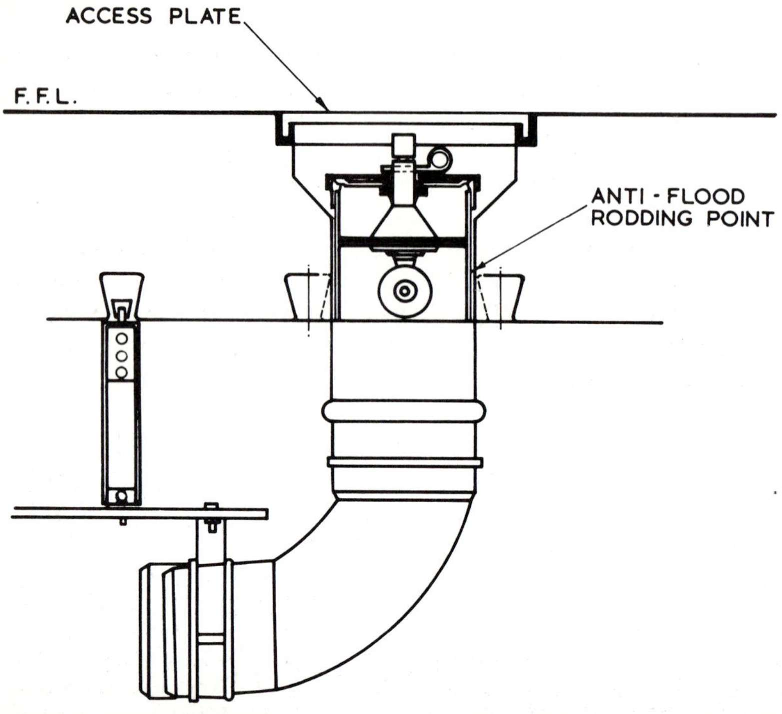

Fig. 11.6 Sealed rodding point

sonal hygiene such as the washing of exposed parts of the body that may get splashed during the cleaning operation, wearing of face masks to prevent inhaling fumes and, in particular, the washing of hands before eating.

Types of maintenance

If the sanitary systems have been correctly designed, properly installed, and are used with discretion, maintenance should be minimal and planned.

Planned maintenance in its simplest form is the cleaning of sanitary equipment and the removal of deposits from traps. In very large buildings such as hospitals it takes the form of a procedure to be undertaken over a twelve-month period and recorded on forms specifically designed for the purpose.

Emergency maintenance is that which is required when, for no known reason, a blockage suddenly occurs within the pipework and effluent appears in unacceptable places. It is sometimes called crisis maintenance and is often associated with very old sanitary systems and/or deliberate or accidental misuse.

Because of the difficulty of access, the maintenance and inspection of flat roof gutters is often not undertaken until evidence of neglect; e.g. when water appears through the ceiling of a room below. Again, an annual inspection is necessary, and the removal of debris from the gutters and outlets carried out. If such outlets become blocked, ponding on the roof will occur and water may find its way into the building via the parapet or roof light flashings.

Water can also enter the roof around the gutter outlet either when the waterproof membrane is poorly fixed into the outlet or when the outlet has moved relative to the roof surface. This is shown in Fig. 11.7 where the outlet was fixed to a vertical length of internal downpipe that had no provision for movement in its total length. Therefore, when the building settled slightly – as all buildings will, due to their weight – the vertical pipe pushed the roof outlet up by approximately 25 mm, forming a pond in the gutter. It also split the felt covering, allowing water to penetrate the roof.

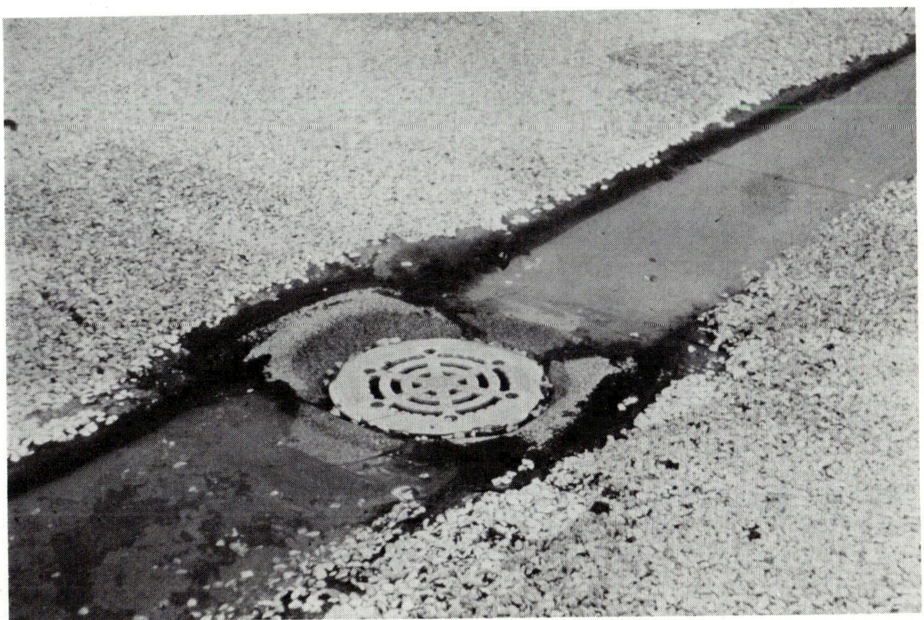

Fig. 11.7 Defective roof outlet junction

Defective rainwater downpipes (and external foul stacks) can cause considerable damage to the structure of a building and can also make the external appearance of a building unsightly. Water leaking from such pipework can penetrate through the wall of solid brickwork and affect the internal plaster work and decorative finish; it can also damage the mortar jointing and bricks. Saturated joints and bricks are easily damaged by the action of frost and expensive repair work on the building will be necessary.

As vertical corrosion cracks at the back of the downpipe are difficult to detect when the pipe is close to the wall face, all external cast iron downpipes should

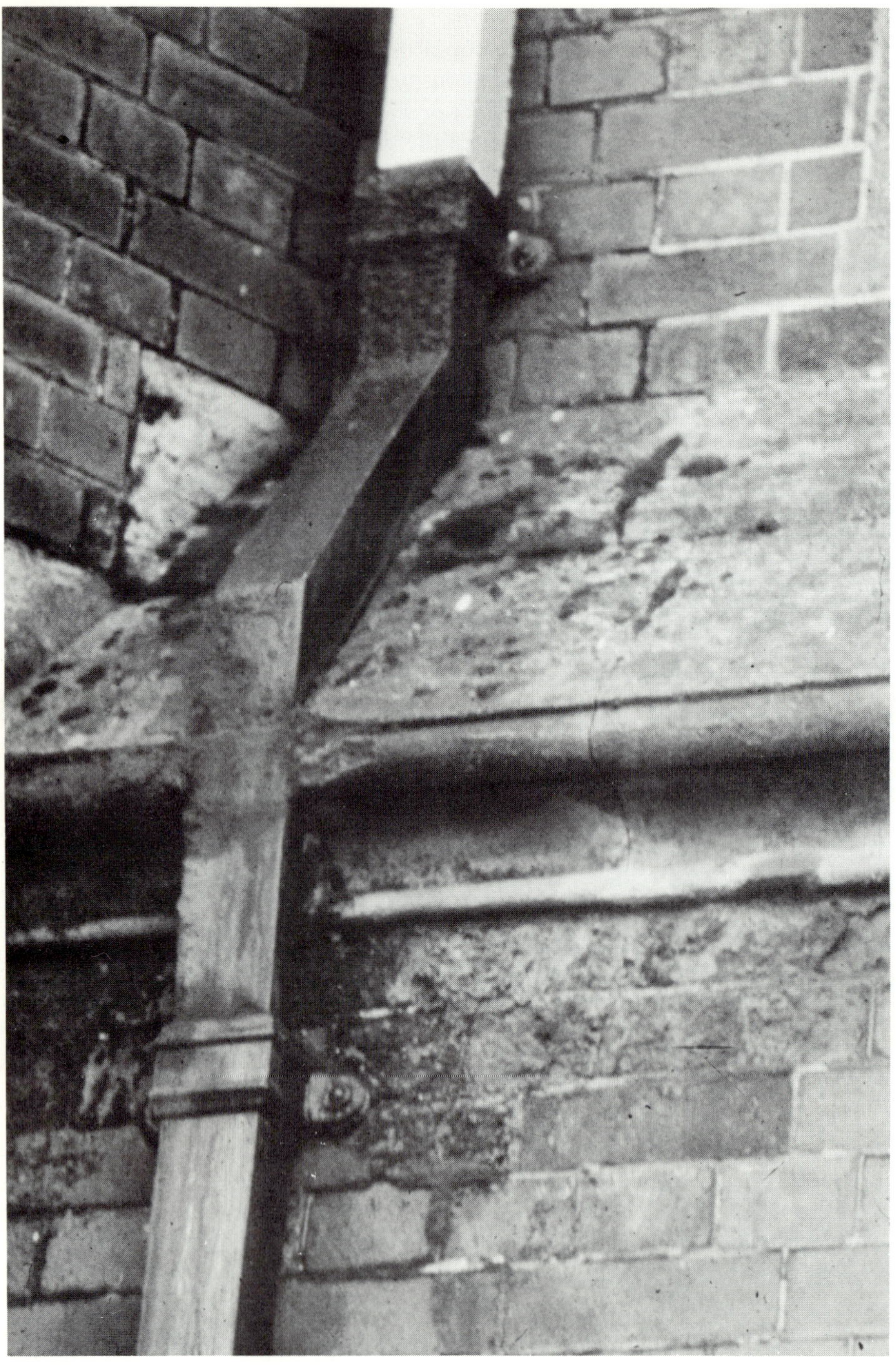

be off the face of the building to allow complete visual annual inspection and to enable painting to be carried out completely around the circumference of the pipe.

If they are not correctly fixed painting is only cosmetic and does not give protection to the back line of the pipe.

PVC external rainwater stacks may be subject to either deliberate or accidental physical damage at ground level; in these cases the bottom section should be replaced by spun iron spaced on lugs to keep it off the wall face.

Planned maintenance

In a large estate or building it is desirable to organize a maintenance programme for the sanitary systems. This programme should cover the internal systems and appliances and the external systems. It can be further sub-divided into the following:

(a) roof drainagc;
(b) foul drainage;
(c) surface water from paved areas, roads and car parks;
(d) subsoil drainage.

The objective of planned maintenance is to keep the systems functioning as required by the user, to prevent them declining in standard due to use and age and to prevent damage or risk to health by the systems failing.

There is no point in maintaining a system that is continuously failing; by which is meant, not functioning as the user requires.

If a part of a system or point in a system can be identified as causing trouble it is better to carry out remedial work rather than continuous maintenance, and it is nearly always more cost effective.

A programme of planned maintenance for the rainwater gutters, flashings and all external stacks should also be the objective of any building estate manager, both to protect his estate from water damage and to keep the systems in good working condition.

As well as the inspections and remedial work quoted it is important that gutters are cleaned out at set intervals and not allowed to become blocked by falling leaves, etc.

Although plastic gutter systems if properly installed require no maintenance against the action of the weather, they will require regular clearing out or they will, in time, become blocked by debris.

Figure 11.10 shows the outline of a building at ground floor level and identifies the manholes, the rodding points and gullies, etc. The building is on a grid so that each maintenance point position can be identified.

Fig. 11.8 (facing page) Square section downpipe

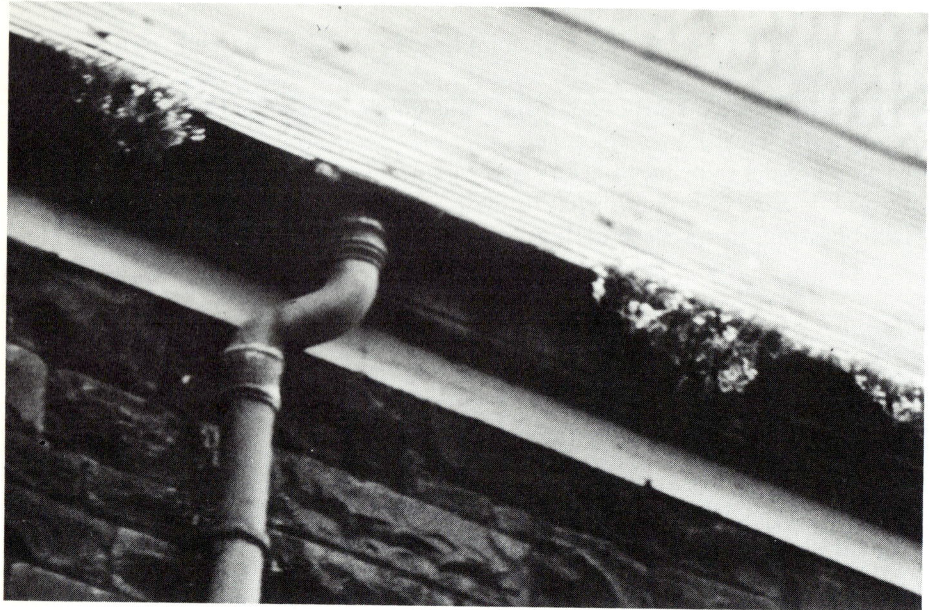

Fig. 11.9 Gutter system blocked by grass

Attached to Fig. 11.10 is a Work Schedule (Fig. 11.11) that gives the work reference as set out in a work programme and the time interval between operations. As well as the work indicated in the Work Schedule it is recommended that an annual visual inspection of the building or estate is undertaken and if the maintenance operator reports that a maintenance point is defective it should be surveyed and remedial work put in hand to prevent a drain failure occurring.

To put in hand a programme based on the above simplified example it is essential that the maintenance manager knows his estate or building. Particularly in old estates, the recorded information is usually out of date, or even non-existent. Reliance cannot be placed upon old drawings that have not been accurately updated.

It is therefore essential when setting up a planned maintenance programme to carry out a survey to record the site drainage systems including all manholes, gullies, etc. These need not be accurately positioned on a drawing, but must be easily identified by the grid system.

The main site record drawing should be to a scale not less than 1 : 500; each building should then be shown on a single sheet of paper to a scale of about 1 : 250 and coupled with a work schedule.

The work manual (Fig. 11.12) should be a simple booklet capable of being understood and used by the maintenance operative.

This system of planned maintenance can be carried out by in-house staff or can be sub-contracted out to a skilled organization. It is, however, essential to

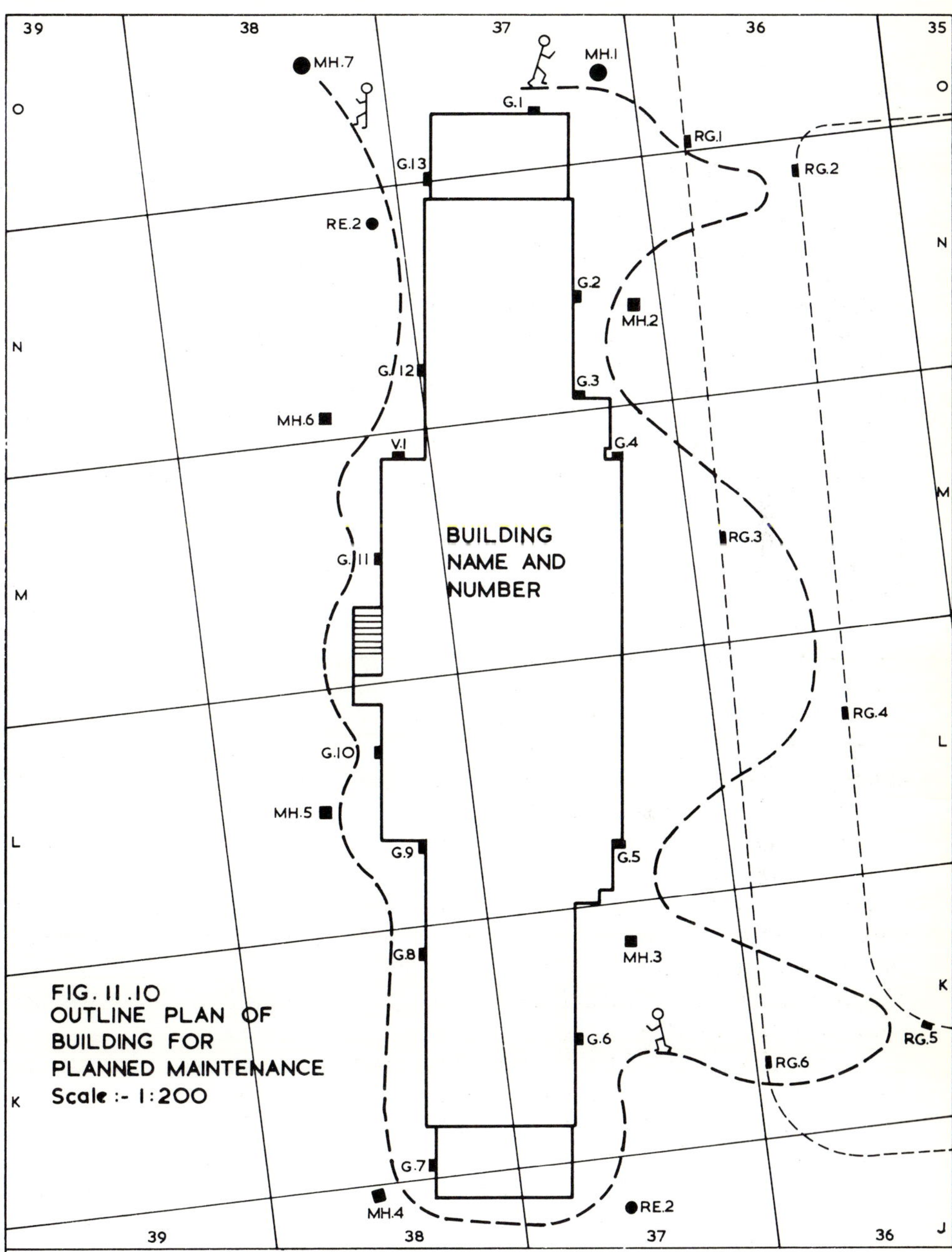

Fig. 11.10 Outline plan of building for planned maintenance

Fig. 11.11 'Work Schedule' for planned maintenance programme

Building name ....
Building No. ....
Drawing No. ....
F – Foul S – Surface water C – Combined

No.	Drain type			Grid	Class	Work operation code	Remarks
	MH no.	Gully no.	road gully no.	ref.			
1	1			37/O	F	A1	Chemical waste
2	2			37/N	F	A1	
3	3			37/K	C	A1	
4	4			38/J	S	A1	
5	5			38/L	C	A1	
6	6			38/N	F	A1	
7	7			38/O	S	A1	
8		1		37/O	F	A2	Chemical waste
9		2		37/N	F	A2	
10		3		37/N	S	A2	
11		4		37/M	F	A2	
12		5		37/L	C	A5	Combined Surface/Foul
13		6		37/K	S	A2	
14		7		38/K	S	A2	
15		8		38/K	F	A2	
16		9		38/L	F	A2	
17		10		38/L	F	A2	
18		11		38/M	C	A5	Combined Surface/Foul
19		12		37/N	F	A2	
20		13		37/O	S	A2	
21			1	36/O	S	A4	
22			2	36/N	S	A4	
23			3	36/M	S	A4	
24			4	36/L	S	A4	
25			5	36/K	S	A4	
26			6	36/K	S	A4	
27					V1	A3	Air vent
28					RE1	A6	Rodding eye
29					RE2	A6	Rodding eye

Fig. 11.12 Example of 'Work Manual'

Work operations
Time intervals between operations:
Y – Yearly;
S – Six monthly;
W – Weekly.

All manholes – Y.
1. Remove cover and clean frame.
2. Inspect cover and frame for defects.
3. Inspect for build-up of solids on benching, etc., clear interceptor trap and flush chamber.
4. Flush drainage connections to manhole and check flows. If there is evidence of grease build-up use degreasing agent. If blockage suspected, rod and report.
5. Inspect step irons for safety and report defects.
6. Inspect for damage or defects:
   (a) Chamber
   (b) Cover slab or reducing slab or taper
   (c) Benching
   (d) Channel
   and report any defects.
7. Grease frame and replace cover.

All gullies – Y
1. Remove grating, clean grating and seating.
2. Clean trap.
3. Flush gully.
4. Check outlet functions correctly, and if there is evidence of grease build-up, flush with degreasing agent.
5. Check waste pipes discharge.
6. Report any defects.

Air vent – Y
1. Check mica flap is in position and free to move.
2. Check pipework is undamaged and free from rubbish.
3. Check condition of paintwork.
4. Report any defects.

Road gullies – Y
1. Clear away debris from grating.
2. Remove grating, clean grating and seating.
3. Clean gully and silt container.
4. Flush with water, if possible.
5. Check outlet functions correctly.
6. Report any defects

Note: Where possible this yearly maintenance should be made to coincide with the end of the leaf fall. More frequent attention may be necessary in certain locations depending upon local conditions.

Combined gullies – S
1. Clear away debris from grating.
2. Remove grating, clean grating and seating.
3. Clean out gully and silt basket if fitted.
4. Flush gully.
5. Check for grease build-up and clean if necessary.
6. Check waste pipes discharging into gully.
7. Check rainwater pipe in side inlet or over gully, clean if required.
8. Test gully that drain is functioning correctly.
9. Report any defects.

Note: Where possible this operation should coincide with annual leaf fall. When in proximity of pine trees and where rubbish may accumulate on the grating more frequent attention may be required.

All rodding eyes – Y
1. Take off and inspect cover and sealing gasket.
2. Flush through 9 litres of cold water.
3. Check for back pressure.
4. Replace cover and renew seal if necessary.
5. Report defects.

---

reduce such maintenance to a minimum by reducing the number of points to be maintained and the number of times annually it is required to carry out their maintenance. An example of this is the use of an open rainwater gully. Such a gully will require maintaining at least once a year, possibly twice a year. If the gully is replaced by a slow bend with rodding facilities no maintenance will be required.

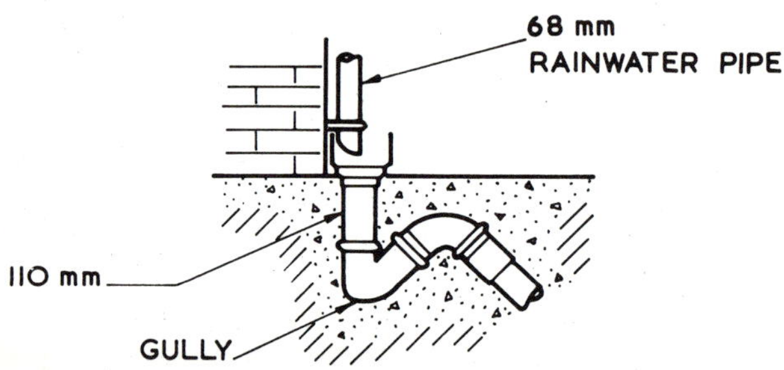

Fig. 11.13 Rainwater shoe and gully

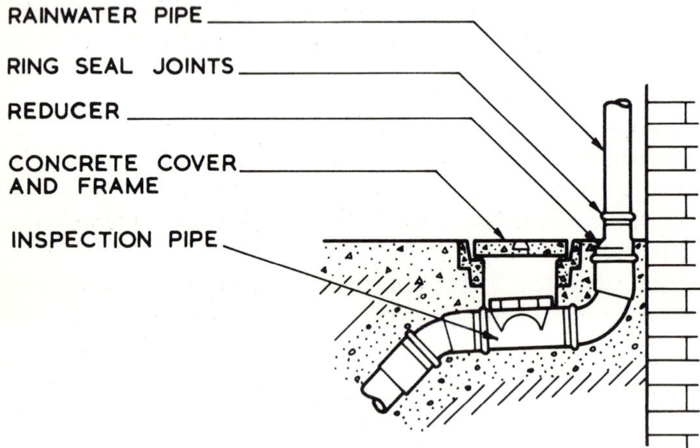

Fig. 11.14 Rainwater direct connection with rodding facilities

Gutters, downpipes and flashings

The maintenance of gutters, downpipes and flashings is just as important as the maintenance of the sanitary systems.

A failure may not create the risks to health that a drain blockage will, but water pouring through the roof can be very inconvenient and can cause considerable damage both to the contents and fabric of the building. In buildings such as long-stay geriatric hospitals it can mean moving all the patients out of the unit before repair work can be carried out.

Gutters, downpipes and flashings should form part of a total planned maintenance programme and should always be visually inspected annually before the onset of winter.

If a defective gutter or donwpipe is left for any length of time water will penetrate the fabric of the building, often necessitating expensive repair work. This type of repair work is always costly as it requires the erection of scaffolding, which in itself can cause a nuisance by blocking the light from windows and the movement of goods and people in the vicinity of the operation.

Defective eaves gutters can allow water to affect both the roof construction and the cladding. The example shown in Fig. 11.9 is a defective joint in an OG cast iron gutter mounted on a moulded timber fascia. When the gutter was inspected it was found that the back had rusted to such a degree that the whole system had to be dismantled and replaced. It was also found that the fascia had been damaged by the water and the ends of the joists were rotten, all requiring expensive repair work.

A close inspection of any cast iron gutter system should be carried out every three to five years depending upon the exposure of the site; repair work should be organized to coincide with the painting of the windows, fascias and gutters, etc. to save repetitive scaffolding.

It has been found that it is more economical to completely take down cast iron OG gutters and replace them by pastic which require less maintenance.

Emergency maintenance

The necessity for such maintenance indicates that there is something wrong with the system or the way the system is being used. The problem is to identify the point of failure and diagnose why it is occurring.

Blockages requiring emergency treatment usually occur at inconvenient times; the first indication of such a blockage is usually a report that sewage or water is flooding from an appliance on to the floor, or is backing up through a gully. If this occurs in a critical area of a building such as a food processing room or kitchen it may be necessary to condemn all the food in the area, and carry out a deep cleaning operation as well as clear the blockage; all this incurs great expense.

A single isolated blockage is usually caused by the misuse of the system; someone flushes through a WC an object that will not clear the system and may lodge on a bend or junction.

If the blockages continue to occur in roughly the same place the reason must be identified and remedial work carried out to eliminate its reoccurrence. A

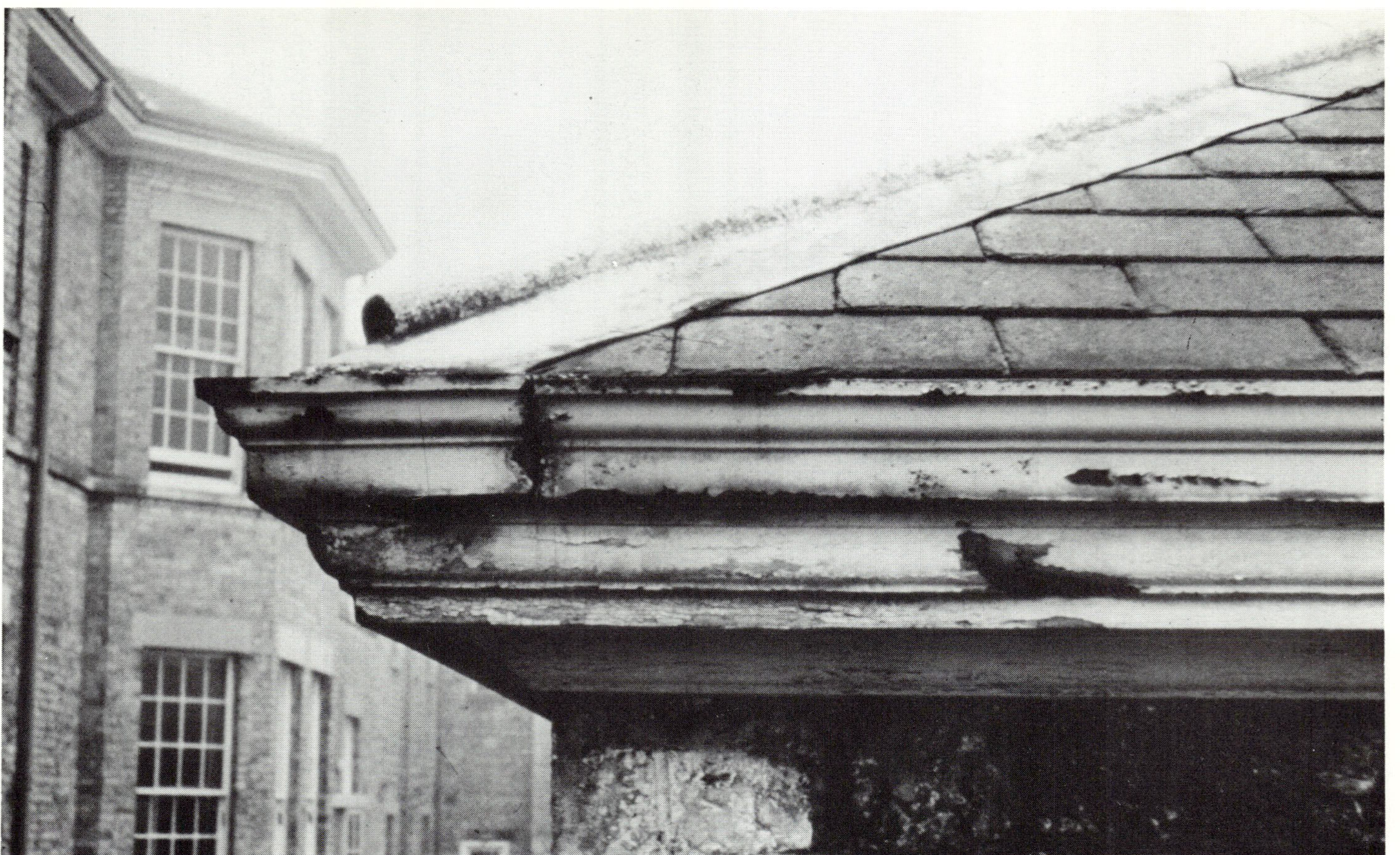

Fig. 11.15 Defective joint in OG gutter

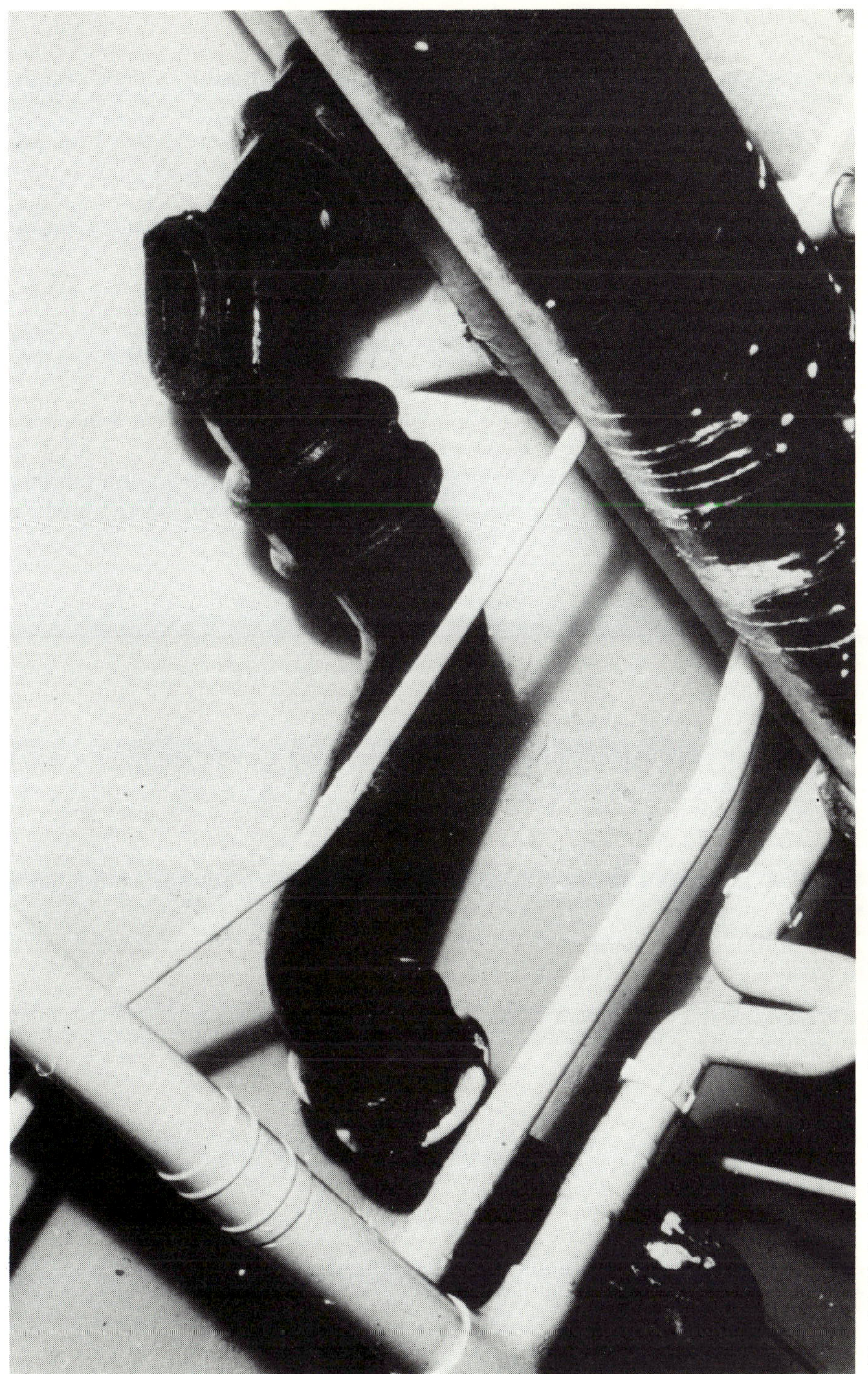

Fig. 11.16 Acute bends cause blockages

typical example is the use of acute bends, possibly with poorly made joints. By the removal of the two bends and their replacement by one large radiused bend of a smooth material and well-made joints the point of trouble will be eliminated.

It is not always possible to carry out remedial work to an existing drainage system. In these cases good management is essential. There is no point in discharging into the system solids that are known to cause blockages, i.e. food waste, paper towels, maternity pads, etc. Other means of disposal must be used, such as bags and incineration.

Again, a survey of the system is essential, both to identify the point of trouble and to ascertain the cause. Sometimes an increase in the water flow will reduce the risk of blockages developing, or the screw fixing of grilles to gullies will prevent the unauthorized disposal of items likely to cause trouble.

The installation of blockage indicators will give early warning that a blockage has occurred before a spillage is noted. These devices can also be wired to solinoid valves which will switch off the water supply to equipment and sanitary appliances such as WCs so they cannot be used, thereby reducing the load on the system.

Equipment

There is available today a wide range of equipment and techniques for carrying out the maintenance of sanitary systems.

Traditionally, maintenance has been carried out by a plumber using a set of cane rods and a rubber plunger; at best he would also have a flexible spiral wire. Maintenance is now a specialist operation and there are many companies operating nationwide willing and able to solve these problems. Some are good, but some not so good, and have been known to cause as much trouble as they have cured.

The equipment available can generally be divided into five categories, each with advantages and disadvantages. They are:

1. Rods and wires.
2. Pressure devices.
3. Water jetters.
4. Drag lines.
5. Chemicals.

Rods and wires

These are similar to the traditional equipment used by the plumber.
In the most basic terms they fall into two types:

(a) Rigid cane or steel rods that will flex to a small degree. Cane or steel sectional rods can be jointed together and manually pushed down a drain pipe to puncture the blockage, thereby allowing the effluent to flow away, hopefully taking the cause with it. These rods cannot negotiate bends or junctions and cannot be pushed very far. The end of the rod can be fitted with a range of tools which may carry out a variety of functions. Within limits this method will work, but often it is the case that the blockage is only punctured and remain fixed in position.

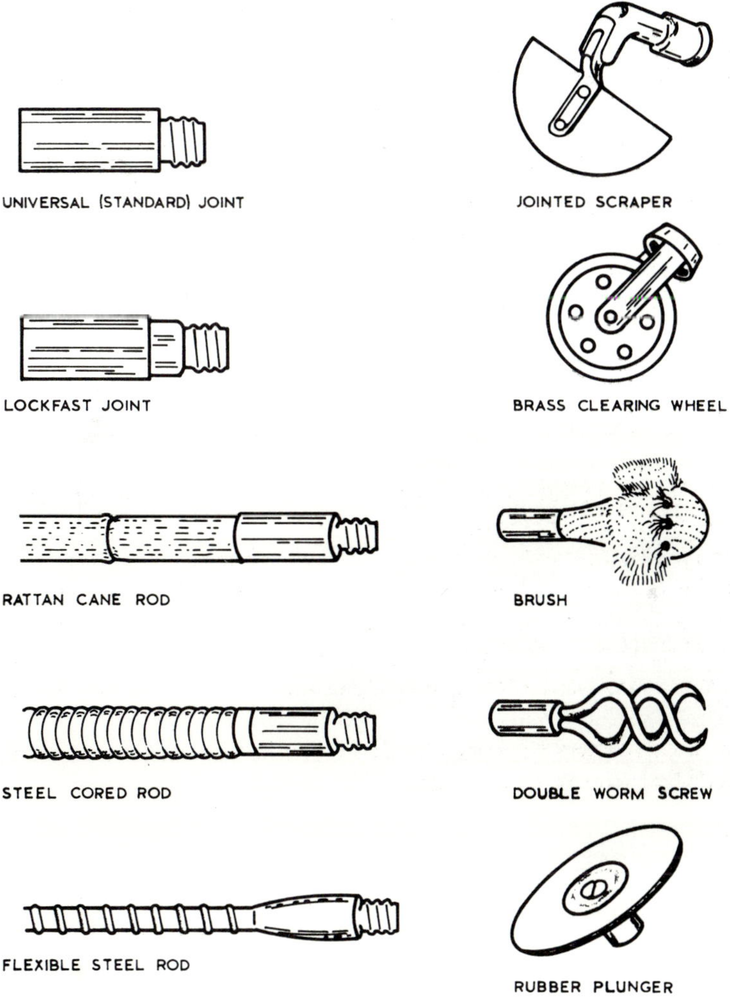

Fig. 11.17 Selection of rods and tools

(b) Hand-operated spiral wires. These have been in existence for a very long time they are usually of small diameter and so flexible that they can negotiate a 'P' or 'S' trap. This type of equipment has been 'modernized' by being power assisted. Wires are spirally wound, of great strength and powered by either electrical or petrol-driven motors. They come in a variety of diameters and lengths and are housed in a drum. The end of the wire is inserted into the drain, can be fitted with a variety of cutting heads and the speed of operation manually controlled. The objective of these power-propelled wires is the same as the cane rods, i.e. to penetrate the drainage system until the head comes to the blockage and then destroy the object causing the trouble. There are a variety of sizes of these devices from a simple electric hand-held wire suitable for use in pipes up to 110 mm in size, to large wheeled petrol driven motorized units capable of working in drains up to 300 mm in diameter.

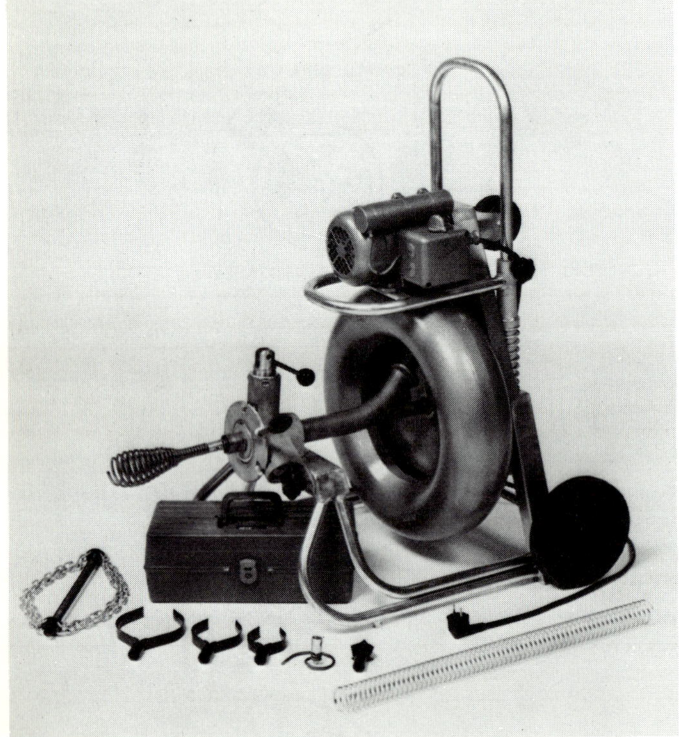

Fig. 11.18 Example of large power assisted wire

Pressure devices

These devices work on the principle that water cannot be compressed, but will transmit a shock wave with little loss of energy if one end of a tube full of water is struck. The most basic example of this is the use of a rubber plunger which, if pushed up and down in a flooded appliance, will create a pressure on the point of the blockage.

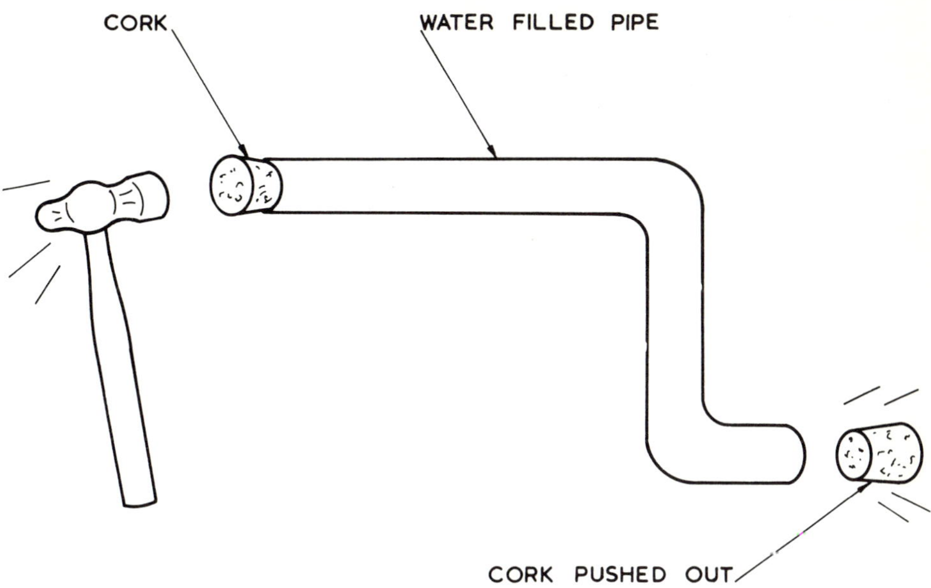

Fig. 11.19 Example of kinetic energy

A more sophisticated product is the kinetic gun, which consists of an air cylinder capable of being charged by either manual pumping or an external source. The gun is directed through the blocked appliance and the air pressure quickly released by a trigger, thereby creating a shock wave to the point of the blockage.

These devices can cause back pressure problems and should only be carefully used after initial training.

They have another practical application, which is the clearing of a partially blocked pipe. By attaching the gun to a running water source which will fill the partially blocked pipe with water the action of releasing the air will scour the pipe and remove sedimentary deposits.

Water jetters

The method of drain cleaning by water jetting is the application of water pressure to firstly get the tool to the blockage and then to remove the source of the trouble.

The equipment takes the form of a pressure pump mounted on a trailer, usually powered by a petrol motor. It has a reel of hose pipe at the leading end of which is a specially designed head with integral jets, some facing forwards and some obliquely backwards.

The object of the backwards-facing jets is two-fold; first, to push the hose through the pipe to be cleaned, and second, to strip off any build-up of deposit on the wall of the pipe. The forward-facing jet is used to cut through the blockage.

This method of drain cleaning is excellent, particularly when access is only through manholes outside a building. It is ideal for the removal of sedimentary deposits in surface water and land drains.

Drag lines

The use of this type of equipment is mainly in very large diameter sewers. The winches can be either hand or power operated and the technique is simple. A wire or rope is passed through the pipe to be cleaned between two access chambers, a winch attached to the rope at one end and a scraper or bucket, etc., attached to the other end and slowly dragged through. A second winch may also be used to draw back the tool. The equipment is often used when sewers sediment up with detritus or grit and have their capacity reduced.

Chemicals

The cleaning of waste pipework by acid drip feeding can sometimes be effective, particularly in the case of lime scale encrustation in urinal wastes. The acid suitable is a 40 per cent solution by mass in water of orthophosphoric acid with surface active agents and corrosion inhibitors.

It must be noted that acid-based cleaners, when in contact with chlorine bleach cleaners, produce chlorine gas, which is toxic, and any toilet accommodation where this method of cleaning is being used must be well ventilated.

Some blockages are caused by an accumulation of grease and soap residues; these can be successfully cleaned by a solution of very hot water with soda crystals added. The recommendation is to fill a basin or sink with very hot water and add 1 kg of soda crystals to every 9 litres of water; when fully dissolved, remove the plug to flush the trap and pipework. This technique may require more than one application.

Caustic soda should not be used in place of soda crystals.

It has been noted that there are a number of organizations promoting the use of chemical agents for drain cleaning, some of which can cause damage to the pipework system and also to the user. One product is based upon 'concentrated sulphuric acid' with an added inhibitor against attacking steel, iron, copper or brass; it is also safe for most plastic systems, but should not come into contact with pitch fibre or rubber compounds.

Another product contains a concentrate of orthodichlorobenzine, which is a solvent de-greaser and pesticide. Poisoning has been reported in man, the main route being absorption through the skin. The toxic effects vary and include dermatitis, pneumonitis, lung granulomata and liver and kidney damage, central nervous system depression and blood disorders.

One can only say that when considering using chemical cleaning methods ensure that the composition of the product is known and checked by the Health and Safety Executive as to its safety in the application being considered.

Reference addresses

Trade associations

Asbestos Cement Manufacturers' Association	c/o Dickens House, 15 Tooks Court London EC4H 1LA 01–242 7161
British Bath Manufacturers' Association	Fleming House, Renfrew Street, Glasgow C3 041–332 0826
British Malleable Tube Fittings Association	St Vedast House, 150 Cheapside, London EC2V 6JA 01–698 8856
British Non-Ferrous Metals Federation	6 Bathurst Street, London W2 2SD 01–723 7465
British Plastics Federation	47/48 Piccadilly London W1 01–734 2041
British Pump Manufacturers' Association	37 Castle Street, Guildford, Surrey GU1 3UQ 0483 37991
British Steel Corporation	P O Box 403, 33 Grosvenor Place London SW1 01–235 1212
British Valve Manufacturers' Association	3 Buckingham Gate, London SW1E 6JH 01–834 1496
British Water & Effluent Treatment Plant Association	27 Crendon Street, High Wycombe, Bucks, HP13 6LG 0494 444 544
Council of British Ceramic Sanitaryware Manufacturers (CBCSM)	Federation House, Stoke-on-Trent, Staffs 0782 48675
Copper Tube Fittings Manufacturers' Association (CTFMA)	7 Highfield Road, Birmingham B15 3ED 021–454 7766
Metal Sink Manufacturers' Association	c/o Chamber of Commerce House P O Box 360, 75 Harborne Road, Birmingham B15 3DH 021–454 6171
National Association of Fire Officers	Palace Chambers, Bridge Street, London SW1 01–839 5011
National Federation of Builders' and Plumbers' Merchants	15 Soho Square, London W1 01–439 1753
Pitch Fibre Pipe Association of Great Britain	35 New Bridge Street, London EC4V 6BH 01–248 5271
Plastic Pipe Manufacturers' Society	c/o Wenham Major & Clarke, 89 Cornwall Street, Birmingham 3 Warwickshire 021–236 1866

Institutes

Architectural Association	36 Bedford Square, London WC1 01-636 0974
Association of Consulting Engineers	Hancock House, 87 Vincent Square London SW1P 2PH 01–222 6557
Association of Local Government Engineers and Surveyors	P O Box No. 628, 37 Wimbledon Hill Road, London SW19 OPF 01-946 377
Association of London Borough Engineers and Surveyors	128–142 High Road, Ilford, Essex IG1 1DD (Ext. 145) 01–478 3020
Association of Water Officers	15 Market Place, South Shields Tyne and Wear NE33 1JQ 089–43 63882
Building Services Engineering Society	c/o The Intitution of Civil Engineers, 1–7 Great George Street, London SW1P 3AA 01–930 7444
Chartered Institution of Building Services	49 Cadogan Square, London SW1 01–235 7671
Council of Engineering Institutions	2 Little Smith Street, London SW1 01–799 3912
Engineers' Registration Board	2 Little Smith Street, Westminster SW1P 3DL 01–799 3912
Incorporated Association of Architects and Surveyors	29 Belgrave Square, London SW1 01–235 3755
The Institution of Clerks of Works of Great Britain Incorporated	41 The Mall, Ealing, London W5 3TJ 01–579 2917
Institute of Plumbing	Scottish Mutual House, 29 North Street Hornchurch RM11 1RU 040 24 51236
Institute of Quantity Surveyors	98 Gloucester Place, London W14 AT 01–935 1859/4048
Institute of Water Pollution Control	Ledson House, 53 London Road, Maidstone Kent ME16 8JH 0622 62034
Institute of Registered Architects	68 Gloucester Place, London W1 01–486 1945
Institution of Chemical Engineers	16 Belgrave Square, London, SW1 01–235 3647
Institution of Civil Engineers	1 Great George Street, London SW1 01-839 3611
Institution of Corrosion Technology	14 Belgrave Square, London SW1X 8PZ 01–245 9189
Institution of Municipal Engineers	25 Eccleston Square, London SW1 01–834 5082
Institution of Public Health Engineers	32 Eccleston Square, London SW1 01–834 3017
Institution of Structural Engineers	11 Upper Belgrave Street, London SW1 01–235 4535
Institution of Water Engineers	6–8 Sackville Street, London W1 01–734 5422
Plastics Institute	11 Hobart Place, London SW1 01–245 9555
Royal Incorporation of Architects in Scotland	15 Rutland Square, Edinburgh 1, Scotland 031–229 7205/6

Royal Institute of British Architects	66 Portland Place, London W1N 4AD 01–580 5533
Royal Institute of Public Health and Hygiene	28 Portland Place, London W1 01–580 2731
Royal Institution of Chartered Surveyors	12 Great George Street, London SW1 01–930 2081
Royal Society for the Promotion of Health	13 Grosvenor Place, London SW1 01–235 9961
Royal Town Planning Institute, The	26 Portland Place, London W1N 4BE 01–636 9107

Research and Advisory Bodies

Agrément Board	Lord Alexander House, Waterhouse Street Hemel Hempstead, Herts Hemel Hempstead 3701
British Cast Iron Research and Development Association	Bordersley Hall, Alvechurch, Worcestershire 073–92 66414
British Iron and Steel Research Association	24 Buckingham Gate, London SW1 01–828 7931
British Non-Ferrous Metals Federation	Crest House, 7 Highfield Road, Edgbaston, Birmingham B15 3ED 021–454 7766
British Standards Institution	2 Park Street, London W1 01–629 9000
Technical Help to: Exporters Department, BSI	Maylands Avenue, Hemel Hempstead, Herts HP2 4SQ. Hemel Hempstead 111
British Steel Corporation Special Steels Division	Alloy & Stainless Steels Works Group P O Box 150, Tinsley Park Works, Sheffield SO 1TQ 074–40311
British Non-Ferrous Metals Technology Centre	Grove Laboratories, Denchworth Road, Wantage, Oxon OX12 9BJ 02357 2992
Building Cost Information Service	85–87 Clarence Street, Kingston-upon-Thames, Surrey KT1 1RB 01–549 2542
Building Maintenance Cost Information Service Ltd	85–87 Clarence Street, Kingston-upon-Thames, Surrey KT1 1RB 01–549 0102/3
Building Research Establishment	Garston, Watford, Herts 09273 74040
Building Research Advisory Service	Building Research Station, Garston, Watford, WD2 7JR Herts 09273 76612
Fire Research Station	Borehamwood, Herts, WD6 2BL 01–953 6177
Princes Risborough Laboratory	Princes Risborough, Aylesbury, Bucks HP17 9PX. Princes Risborough 084 44 3101
BRE Scottish Laboratory	Kelvin Road, East Kilbride, Glasgow G75 0RZ. 035 52 33941
Building Services Research and Information Association (BSRIA)	Old Bracknell Lane, Bracknell, Berks RG12 4AH. 0344 25071
Construction Industry Research and Information Association	Old Queen Street House, 6 Storey's Gate, London, SW1 01–839 6881

Copper Development Association (CDA)	Orchard House, Mutton Lane, Potters Bar, Herts 0707 50711
Fire Offices' Committee	Aldermary House, Queen Street, London EC4N 1TJ 01–248 5222
Fire Research Station	Melrose Avenue, Borehamwood, Herts. 01–953 6177
Hydraulics Research Station	Wallingford, Berkshire 059–13 2381
Lead Development Association	34 Berkeley Square, London W1X 6AJ 01–499 8422
National Building Agency	NBA House, Arundel Street, London WC2 01–836 4488
National House-Builders Council	58 Portland Place, London W1N 4BU 01–387 7201

Building Centres, The Association of London:

London:	
The Building Centre	26 Store Street, London, WC1E 7BT 01–637 1022
(Administration):	(Information) 01–637 9001
	(Bookshop) 01–637 3151
Birmingham:	
Engineering and Building Centre	Broard Street, Birmingham B1 2DB 021–643 1914
Coventry:	
Coventry Building Information Centre	Council House, Earl Street, Coventry, CV1 5SE 0203 25555 Ext. 2512
Bristol:	
The Building Centre, Bristol	Colston Avenue, The Centre, Bristol BS1 4TW.
	(Information) 0272 27002
	(Administration) 0272 22953
Cambridge:	
The Building Centre, Cambridge	15–16 Trumpington Street, Cambridge CB2 1QD 0223 59625
Stoke-on-Trent:	
The Building Information Centre	College of Building and Commerce Stoke Road, Shelton, Stoke-on-Trent, ST4 2DG 0782 24651
Glasgow:	
The Building Centre, Scotland	6 Newton Terrace, Glasgow G3 7PF 041–248 6212
Liverpool:	
Building and Design Centre	Hope Street, Liverpool L1 9BR
	(Information) 051–709 8484
	(Administration) 051–709 8566
Manchester:	
The Building Centre, Manchester	113–115 Portland Street Manchester, M1 6FB.
	(Information) 061–236 6933
	(Administration) 061–236 9802

Nottingham: Midland Design and Building Centre	Mansfield Road, Nottingham NG1 3FE 0602 45651
Southampton: The Building Centre, Southampton	Grosvenor House, 18–20 Cumberland Place, Southampton S01 2BD. 0703 27350
Building Centre of Ireland	17 Lower Baggot Street, Dublin 2 Dublin 762745

Advisory and research bodies

National Water Council	1 Queen Anne's Gate, London SW1H 9BT 01–930 3100
NWC Testing Station	The Causeway, Staines, Middlesex TW 18 3DR 0784–54626
Plastics and Rubber Institute	11 Hobart Place, London SW1 01–245 9555
Royal Society of Health	90 Buckingham Palace Road, London SW1 01–730 5134
Rubber and Plastics Research Association	Shawbury, Shrewsbury 5YR 4NR 093–94 383
Steel Sheet Information and Development Association	Albany House, Petty France, London SW1 01–799 1616
Town and Country Planning Association	17 Carlton House Terrace, London SW1Y 5AS 01–930 8903/4/5
Vitreous Enamel Development Council Ltd.	28 Welbeck Street, London W1M 7PG 01-486 2237
Water Research Centre	Ferry Lane, Medmenham, Marlow, Bucks. 049–166 531
Welding Institute	Abington Hall, Abington, Cambridge 0223–891162

Regional water authorities and water companies in England and Wales

North West Water Authority	Dawson House, Great Sankey, Warrington Lancs WA5 3LW Penketh 092 572 4321
South West Water Authority	3–5 Barnfield Road, Exeter, EX1 1RE 0392 50861
Yorkshire Water Authority	West Riding House, 67 Albion Street, Leeds LS1 5AA 0532 448201
Water companies York Waterworks Company	Lendal Tower, Yorks, Y01 2DL 0904 22171
Severn Trent Water Authority	Abelson House, 2297 Coventry Road, Sheldon, Birmingham, B26 3PS 021 743 4222

Water companies	
East Worcestershire Waterworks Co	47 New Road, Bromsgrove, B60 2JT 0527 75151
South Staffordshire Waterworks	50 Sheepcote Street, Birmingham B16 8AR 021–643 8131
Cheadle Water Works Co., Ltd.	43 Chapel Street, Cheadle, Staffordshire Cheadle 05384 2388
Anglian Water Authority	Diploma House, Grammar School Walk, Huntingdon PE18 6NZ 0480 56181
Water companies	
Cambridge Water Company	Rustat Road, Cambridge CB1 3QS 0223 47351
East Anglian Water Company	163 High Street, Lowestoft 0502 2406
Essex Water Company	342 South Street, Romford, Essex RM1 2AL 0708 46706
Tendring Hundred Waterworks Co.	Mill Hill, Manningtree, Essex CO11 2AZ 0206 39 2155
Northumbrian Water Authority	Northumbria House, Regent Centre, Gosforth, Newcastle-Upon-Tyne NE3 3PX 0632 843151
Water companies	
Hartlepools Water Company	3 Lancaster Road, Hartlepool, Co Durham TS24 8LW 0429 4405/6
Newcastle and Gateshead Water Co	P O Box 10, Allendale Road, Newcastle-Upon-Tyne, NE6 2SW 0632 654144
Sunderland and South Shields Water Company	29 John Street, Sunderland SR1 1JT 0783 57123
Southern Water Authority	Guildbourne House, Worthing, Sussex BN11 1LD 0903 205252
Water companies	
Eastbourne Waterworks Company	14 Upperton Road, Eastbourne, Sussex BN21 1EP Eastbourne 0323 21371
Folkstone and District Water Company	The Cherry Garden, Cherry Garden Lane, Folkstone, Kent CT19 9QB 0303 76951
Mid Kent Water Company	P O Box 45, High Street, Snodland, Kent ME6 4AH 240313
Mid Sussex Water Company	6 Boltro Road, Haywards Heath, Sussex RH16 1BA 0444 2662
Portsmouth Water Company	Brockhampton Springs, P O Box No. 8, West Street, Havant, Hants P09 1LG 070 12 6333
West Kent Water Company	Cramptons Road, Sevenoaks, Kent TN14 5DG 0732 52307
Welsh National Water Development Authority	Cambrian Way, Brecon, Powys LD3 7HP 0874 3181
Water companies	
Chester Waterworks Company	15 Newgate Street, Chester CH1 1DR 0244 20501
Wrexham and East Denbighshire Water Company	21 Egerton Street, Wrexham LL11 1ND 0978 2259

Organisation	Address	Telephone
Thames Water Authority	New River Head, Rosebery Avenue, London EC1R 4TP	01–278 2300
Water companies		
Colne Valley Water Company	Blackwell House, Aldenham Road, Watford WD2 2EY	0923 23333
East Surrey Water Company	London Road, Redhill, Surrey RH1 1LJ	0737 66333
Lee Valley Water Company	P O Box 48, Bishop's Rise, Hatfield, Herts A10 9HL	070 72 64311
Mid Southern Water Company	Frimley Green, Camberley, Surrey GU16 6HZ	025 16 503117
North Surrey Water Company	The Causeway, Staines, Middlesex TW18 3BX	0784 55464
Rickmansworth and Uxbridge Valley Water Company	Batchworth, Rickmansworth, Herts WD3 1LB	092 37 76633
Sutton District Water Company	41 Carshalton Road, Sutton, Surrey SM1 4LQ	01-643 8050
Wessex Water Authority	Techno House, Redcliffe Way, Bristol BS1 6NY	0272 25491
Water companies		
Bournemouth and District Water Company	Alderney Waterworks, West Howe, Bournemouth BH11 8NB	020 16 2261
Bristol Waterworks Company	P O Box No. 218, Bridgwater Road, Bristol BS99 7AU.	0272 665881
West Hampshire Water Company	Knapp Mill, Mill Road, Christchurch, Dorset BH23 2LU	020 15 3361
The Weld Estate	Lulworth Castle, Dorset	092 941 352
The Cholderton and District Water Company	Estate Office, Cholderton, Salisbury, Wilts	098 064 203

Government departments

Organisation	Address	Telephone
Department of Education and Science	Elizabeth House, York Road, London SE1 7PH	01–928 9222
Department of Employment	8 St James' Square, London SW1	01–930 6200
Department of the Environment	2 Marsham Street, London SW1P 3EB	01–212 3434
Directorate General Water Engineering	2 Marsham Street, London SW1P 3EB	01–212 4014
Building Regulations, Prof. Division	Beckett House, Lambeth Palace Road, London SE1	01–928 7855
Property Services Agency: Technical Library	Room C001/C002 Whitgift Centre, Wellesley Road, Croydon CR9 3LY	01–686 8710 + 4560/4564
Building Information Room	Room 1643 Lunar House, Wellesley Road, Croydon CR9 2EL	01–686 3499 + 33060/61
Department of Health and Social Security	Alexander Fleming House, Elephant and Castle, London SE1	01–407 5522

Her Majesty's Stationery Office	Atlantic House, Holborn Viaduct, London EC1 01–248 9876
Meteorological Office	284 High Holborn, London WC1 01–836 4311
Ministry of Agriculture, Fisheries and Food	Whitehall Place, London, SW1 01–839 7711
Scottish Development Department	St Andrew's House, Edinburgh 1 031–556 8501

Training bodies

City and Guilds of London Institute	76 Portland Place, London W1 01–580 3050
Joint Industry Board for Plumbing and Mechanical Engineering Services in England and Wales	Brook House, Brook Street, St Neots Huntingdon, Cambs, PE19 2BP 0480 76925–8
National Joint Council for the Building Industry	11 Weymouth Street, London W1 01–580 1740
Scottish and Northern Ireland Joint Industry Board for Plumbing, Mechanical Engineering Services	2 Walker Street, Edinburgh 031–225 6842/3

Safety organizations

British Safety Council	62/64 Chancellors Road, London W6 9RS 01–741 1231
Health and Safety Executive	Baynards House, 1–13 Chepstow Place, Westbourne Grove, London W2 01–229 3456
Institution of Industrial Safety Officers	23 Queen Square, London WC1N 3AZ 01–278 1796
London Construction Safety Group H M. Govt	Training Centre, Bilton Way, Enfield Middlesex 01–804 2756
Merseyside and North West Safety Centre	c/o Government Training Centre, Stopgate Lane, Aintree, Liverpool L9 6AW 051–525 0702
RoSPA Industrial Safety Training Centre	22 Sumner Road, Acocks Green, Birmingham 27 021–706 4108
Royal Society for the Prevention of Accidents (RoSPA)	Terminal House, 52 Grosvenor Gardens, London SW1 01–730 2246
St John's Ambulance Association and Brigade	1 Grosvenor Crescent, London SW1 7EF 01–235 5231
Yorkshire Safety Section for the Construction Industry	Davidson House, Hales Road, Leeds 12 0532 639227

Index